EMOTION BUFFERS
QUALITY IN HEALTH CARE

EMOTION BUFFERS QUALITY IN HEALTH CARE

Larry M. Hynson, Jr., Ph.D

Associate Professor
Department of Sociology
Oklahoma State University

Ishiyaku EuroAmerica, Inc.
St. Louis • Tokyo

Editor: Gregory Hacke, D.C.

Copyright 1990 by Ishiyaku EuroAmerica, Inc.

Ishiyaku EuroAmerica, Inc.
716 Hanley Industrial Court, St. Louis, Missouri 63144

Library of Congress Catalogue Card Number 90-080093

Hynson, Jr. , Larry M.
  Emotion Buffers: Quality in Health Care

ISBN 0-912791-73-X

Ishiyaku EuroAmerica, Inc.
St. Louis • Tokyo

Composition by The Opticomm Group
St. Louis, Missouri
Printed in the United States of America

Contents

Foreword

AIDS is blitzing the human race like a global hurricane, having uprooted in its wake all aspects of emotions touched by its presence. Behavior has already been indelibly altered, and it can be expected to continue its shift for the foreseeable future under the deadly force of this new disease.

Rarely has an epidemic placed such a biologically focused disease, with concomitant intense emotional stresses, on the specific age segment of our population most free of fatal disease—the 15 through 40-year-olds. This population segment is the most unconditioned to accept fatal disease as an expected feature of life; in contrast, emotional acceptance of death among the elderly is modulated by a degree of rational death expectancy. But this is not so for 15 to 40-year-old people in the prime of life; and as would be expected, emotional stresses associated with this disease are severe and complex.

While the AIDS epidemic gives timely urgency to this text, the general usefulness of this text is for health workers and the interested general public as they try to understand the dynamics of behavior in response to disease. The real usefulness of this text encompasses its application to the entire population in all circumstances wherein the occurrence of disease of any sort invariably stresses the afflicted and their emotional balance in predictable fashion.

Emotional risks are experienced not only in reaction to, but also in living with, devastating disease occurrences. Such diseases can shake the foundation of lives, disrupting an intensely broad range of emotions. Sometimes these intensities of destruction prompt people to contemplate or to commit suicide. But more frequently, the emotional tremblers are much less devastating, so that with some support, people can once again refocus their lives and determine their effectiveness.

Emotions, along with instincts, learned and incorporated values, and knowledge, work together as forces that when combined define and drive our will. These are the forces that cause us to move or act, energizing our attitudes and behavior. Emotions, being derived from our perceptions and fantasies of pleasure and pain, are most vulnerable to the impacts of disease. This vulnerability stems from the fact that emotions, for the most part, operate at unconscious levels. They evolve from, and find expression in, the rather nebulous condition identified as "fear, hate, insecurity, worthlessness, and loneliness."

It is in response to diseases or altered health conditions (perceived, threatened, actual) that a clear understanding of emotional interaction and buffeting behavior is essential for good management practices. This interaction and buffeting behavior can be prescribed and then applied by health care professionals—doctors, nurses, dentists, social workers, and physical therapists—to name but a few. In turn, it is when diseases inevitably occur in all of our lives that a good understanding of emotion buffers can affect our responses to both stress and buffeting and can guide us in making optimal adjustments to prevailing circumstances. That is the message.

The epidemiological dynamics of emotion buffers in health are considered in this text, but health promotion is the ultimate goal. Good practice of medicine is preventive and implies that the general population is prepared for diseases or disasters. That means that individuals who themselves become patients know both how to cope with their emotional responses to crises and, at least throughout any disease or disability event, how to assure the greatest rehabilitation possible in any circumstance. This text should benefit both health professionals in providing better service to patients and the health-minded individuals in improving their understanding of emotions in health and disease.

Daniel J. Schneider, M.D., M.P.H.
Professor and Chairman
Department of Biostatistics and Epidemiology
College of Public Health-University of Oklahoma
January 3, 1989

Preface

Emotion Buffers: Quality in Health Care—"What an unusual book title," you might say. But before you commit yourself, you probably want to know 1) "What exactly does the title mean?" and 2) "How will reading about people's emotions improve my social skills?" The "What is it?" and "How can I use it?" questions should trigger not only your initial reactions as you begin the book, but also your continued responses as you finish the book. From start to finish, these same two questions guided the writing. So what is there about the social dynamics of emotions which, when applied to health care, improves the quality of life? It is simply this: supportive people buffer patients from the harmful effects of stress. With the emotions of patients buffered, that insulation reduces further discouragement and increases quality of life.

The more impersonal the relationship between patient and health care specialists, the more likely the dissatisfaction and malpractice suits when things go bad. If only for that reason alone, the health professional should find this book quite relevant in his, or her, professional pursuits. So as your eyes move across and down the pages, your mind can readily move back and forth in time to confirm either what you already know or how you plan to use this dimension of health care. However, before you read about specific issues and applications, it will help if you realize what this book is not.

This book is neither about brain impairment, nor about the emotional stages of organic mental disorder. It has little to say about the classical psychiatric conditions, and nothing on organic diseases where patients' moods shift radically. Those subjects, about people with extreme emotional states, are left for others so trained. In this book, the subject of health care is seen from a behavioral perspective, a viewpoint that can contribute to quality health care.

The title, therefore, reflects an unusual topic: a different look at human emotions and intervention strategies, an approach which reveals and enhances the need for quality health care. The need for such a look rests on this fundamental premise: high-tech specialties, malpractice law suits, and soaring medical costs limit the personal touch between provider and recipient. Paradoxically, this trend occurs at a time when studies demonstrate how social support enhances quality care. Timely studies of behavioral scientists, nursing researchers, and community mental health clinicians should enhance the climate for quality health care, in spite of the economic upheavals. There is a need to see suffering and ailing humanity from another perspective, and that demands creative exploration: new models, practical thinking, broader analysis, open minds, and a different perspective. If this premise is true, then new insights should help. Our search begins with those disciplines that study human behavior. It is argued that recent sociological research on the social characteristics of emotions has direct application for the Health Sciences.

This book does not, however, elaborate the narrowly defined views of one discipline on emotions. This proposal charts new ground by synthesizing the findings in clinical and field settings with those of academic sociology. Clinical and therapeutic insights about human emotions add to our understanding of people. Experiences in community disaster and/or personal crises confirm the important place of emotions. But these observations can go further and become more useful when combined with certain theoretical underpinnings. The least traveled course is to follow those researchers who examine emotions in a social context. The sociology of emotions becomes the platform for launching specific diagnostic and intervention strategies.

The sociological perspective is defined as a way of looking at broad trends and biographical data. Since human emotions spring from social roots and daily patterns of interaction, that perspective should contribute to theory development. When combined with clinical practice, we have a comprehensive picture of what's happening. Throughout this book, human emotions form the basis for nearly all the writing; including theories, case studies, and practice. This approach is in contrast to the narrow, limited analyses so common in most professional books. Here we examine emotions both in the broader social context and in the narrower individual setting.

Given such broad-based application for the health profession, this book is appropriately divided into three progressively integrated topics. Part One, "Recognizing the Social Context of Emotions," lays the foundation for constructing a sociology of emotions. Several topics discussed in this first division are "The Emotional Side of Health Care," "Tracking Emotions in Self and Society," and "An Integrated Theory of Emotions." Professionals can use these topics to become more aware of the social context of emotions. Freud recognized this association by observing how early experiences influence how people see the world. What begins also continues; friends or family can give stability in crisis. So can strangers with similar experiences.

Part Two is "Identifying the Emotional Dynamics." Topics include: "Sociological Descriptions of Emotions," "Destructive and Constructive Outlets," and "Emotive Analysis and Therapy." Obviously, emotional stability or instability must be interpreted in light of current experiences, especially as a means of overcoming unhealthy emotional states.

Part Three, "Utilizing Emotional Intervention," elaborates the implications. Several case studies validate the need for blending theory and practice in such chapter titles as "The Resource of Personal Encounters," "Intervention Strategies During Recovery," and "Healthy Rediscovery of Dreams." So these three major divisions and their respective chapters present the reader with a broad perspective on emotions. Practitioners can then integrate and apply this perspective to their other strategies.

These topics should appeal to four professional and one non-professional group. The book should interest those directly involved in patient care: nurses (RN, LPN, NA, clinical, specialties), physical and occupational therapists, emergency medical technicians, child life specialists, social workers, medical records personnel, and intake counselors. Interest wanes, however, if the material is presented in the usual heavy style of most scientific texts, journal articles, lab manuals, and hospital handbooks. This book tries to avoid that heavy style by blending facts and illustrations, statistics and examples, theories and applications. So it doesn't matter whether you have taken courses in psychology, human relations, social psychology, or sociology, you can read and understand this book.

Since this book focuses on emotions in health care, it should appeal to a second group: educators concerned about balancing technological training with human understanding. These educators should note the developmental sequence of emotions. Regardless of the educational setting, this text covers a general theme. Whether the students study human behavior, institutional behavior, or field work methods; whether the setting is in a traditional hospital, vocational school, medical school, a clinic, health care facility, community college or university, this book should meet their needs. To these professionals, educators and supervisors, this book clearly departs from the standard book which tends to ignore the emotional dynamics of human predicaments and social problems. When supplemented with your lectures, this text allows students to get a better picture of their chosen profession.

A third group who can benefit from these insights on emotions are those who have studied emotions the most. I am referring to physicians, psychiatrists, psychotherapists, clinical psychologists, mental health technicians, educational therapists, psychiatric so-cial workers, and school health educators who often seek additional insights and approaches for their practice. Even though these professionals already use many other intervention strategies, they continually seek new insights about their clients, especially those patients experiencing social chaos.

And finally, this topic should be read by a fourth group: those professionals found at disasters and emergencies. Included are civil defense workers, Red Cross relief workers, police officers, fire-men, and rescue workers. Some of these disaster workers are not full time professionals, yet they volunteer much of their time and energy. This lay group also includes the informed, intellectual public who read health-related books. After reading this particular book, they should be better informed about normal and abnormal responses to crises.

This book uses the emotions of patients or clients as the common thread for pulling diverse writings together. Other threads such as crisis, emergencies, and disasters could be used, but emotions seem to be the common feature of all tragedies, illnesses, and injuries. When those at the scene of an accident or those in emergency rooms intervene, they see the emotional side of life that few other professionals do.

Traditionally, the Preface contains expressions of indebtedness to those who have contributed significantly to the book's development. To recognize all such people would be impossible; however, there are two groups—high school and university students—to whom I am indebted. Early in my career I served as a Director of Counseling and Guidance and counseled adolescents at a private boarding school. Working with young people broadened my understanding of life changes and emotional responses. Sociological studies confirm what I observed, their move from home to a total institutional setting disrupts established patterns. Subsequent emotional adjustment, however, varies with the degree of social support. Some students were buffered by strong family support and newly established friendships; others were not.

Since 1974, I have supervised hundreds of Oklahoma State University interns placed in social service agencies, hospitals, community-based volunteer groups, support groups, correctional institutions, mental health clinics, prisons, government agencies, and industry. Finding appropriate placements for university students means getting out of the classroom and going into the "real world" where incumbents work. I have interacted with health professionals at Mayo Clinic, The University of Oklahoma Health Sciences Center, Hillcrest Medical Hospital, Tulsa Psychiatric Mental Health Clinic, City of Faith, St. Francis Hospital, and

Children's Medical Center. In addition to conducting professional seminars and training, I also advise students on their placement and work experience. From these experiences I have become more sensitive to health care issues and current intervention strategies.

Although each experience is an individual one, everyone shows some emotions. In unfamiliar settings, a student discovers fears and how to adjust to them. A typical student expresses his anxiety this way: "Suppose I don't do well on the job, what happens then?" As a group, their idealism gives way to the realism of formal organizations. They soon recognize turf disputes, faction groups, attacks on people's integrity and self-esteem. The social support they receive correlates significantly with their adjustment. If their supervisors are positive, they benefit from "self fulfilling prophecy" in which expectations determine much of the outcome.

Regardless of their experiences, which for the most part are quite positive, these students are marginal actors in a competitive drama. Their emotions fluctuate about as much as the recipients or providers in the wards. Observing these young professionals develop has increased my appreciation for the neglected role of human emotions in health care. In our impersonal world, personal sentiments often don't count, or else they're manipulated. Perhaps you've felt that way too. Then these ideas should be of value as they prompt us to be more sensitive to others and how they feel.

I learned something about emotions from these young adults as I observed their emotions during change, crisis, and development. More importantly, I have been exposed to many clinical practices and their respective philosophies. By means of firsthand accounts and face-to-face interaction, I've seen the most recent diagnostic and intervention strategies. Many of these insights, observations, and practices are found in the following pages. It is altogether proper that I dedicate this book to these same young people from whom so many insights and early interests have come. I hope others can now gain from these experiences, experiences which combine theories of classroom learning with the encounters of real life problems.

Introduction

After extended illnesses, patients never fully solve their emotional (and possibly even their physical) problems until they start substituting positive feelings that are socially generated for debilitating ones that rob them of their energy. People need supportive people to find relief from emotional pressures in our society. If that assumption is valid, then we must ask other questions: How does that process work? Who contributes most to the emotional turnaround of depressed patients? Do the same principles operate in community disasters? Car wrecks? Cases of abuse? Implicitly, these are the types of questions asked in the chapters to follow. This introduction sets forth some basic assumptions about medical models, the education process, and treatment strategies—assumptions which need elaboration.

This book focuses on the social dynamics which evolve between patients and providers. Those interpersonal dynamics have implications for health care professionals. Specifically, we will explore how health providers can "plug into" these dynamics. At the crisis, providers become emotion buffers. After the crisis, they sustain social support by training others in the dynamics of empowerment. Social research demonstrates one fact: significant supporters can serve as conduits of emotionally heightened states. They keep the fluctuations of emotions from getting worse, and that is a valuable function, even if it may not contribute directly to patients' physical improvement. In later chapters, we'll examine research on quality of life as it correlates with quality in health care. The central question and ultimate issue is this: Do supportive people provide emotion buffers which allow the stressed an outlet, both for the release of frustrating emotions and the rebuilding of fragmented ones? Practical details come later, but the social dimensions of emotion buffers for health care institutions and providers are briefly stated here in this introduction.

Quality service is not dictated by hospital administrators, it is creatively developed just as social relationships are developed in strong families. Nurses, technicians, and intake counselors can improve quality care when they view themselves as emotion buffers for the distressed. Patients with emotional overloads need supporters to help them absorb the weight of their perplexing pain. In the process, supporters infuse vitality into their patients. Communication among professionals, patients, and friends supplements treatment strategies. Informed consent has more than a healing quality; it also decreases law suits. In 1983, informed consent figured in 28 percent of all medical malpractice law suits, totaling 560 million dollars.

Everyone knows that quality health care at least partly affects quality of life, but not everyone realizes that in times of crisis patients and their families drop the word "partly" from their discussion. During a crisis, quality health care merges into quality of life. As the following chapters emphasize, the proper utilization of emotions in patients may contribute to physical recovery. Professionals who mix trained competency with practical sensitivity recognize the difference between a highly motivated patient and one that is depressed. Professionals respond appropriately. They contribute to this healing because they combine the social art of professional care with the natural science of laboratory competence.

In some health care fields, the psychosocial dimensions are considered real (they are there) but relatively unimportant byproducts of illnesses. Reservations about this topic do exist, but even taking those into account, many social analysts believe that people's "pent up frustrations" probably account for many of today's most pressing health care issues. Peter Reich and Malcom Rogers, both medical professors at Harvard Medical School, believe that "the role of social support in protecting the individual from the effects of stress has been demonstrated....Those who lacked social and community ties were more likely to die of all causes by a factor of almost three."

At a more intense level, emergency medical personnel at Chicago's Westside Hospital watch the Saturday night victims much as they would view some modern horror film. The batterings they observe seem to spring from the screen of their victims' social environment as full-grown emotional nightmares. These bad dreams regularly manifest themselves in the emergency rooms and teaching hospitals of our violent society.

This is not to say that most recognizable causes of illness (germs, microscopic organisms, parasites, infections) go undetected, because they do not. With today's technology, the slightest variations in human cells can be readily detected, accurately diagnosed, and properly treated with amazing precision. Consequently, more and more diseases, along with death itself, are pushed back in time. One frontier remains, however, and it continues to haunt the moderns as much as the ancients. A still unresolved mystery is why people choose a life style which predictably results in so much destruction of bodies, minds, and emotions. It seems that the answer must come, not from isolated efforts, but rather from integrated investigations. The lack of long-term patient compliance seems to be closely correlated with a certain "borderline personality disorder. In many cases, impaired family dynamics, magical hopes for cure, and resentment of physicians for not providing such cures lay beneath the noncompliant behavior" (Roger and Reich, 1988:411).

Cross-fertilization of ideas promotes creativity in health care. The less professionals know about other types of human responses (other than those which they are trained to know), the more dependent they are on their own discipline's orientation. That is a sound strategy for research and for understanding one's professional journals, but it becomes somewhat problematic in health care. The final consideration in health care is the patient, not the purity of a discipline. Those in patient care find it more difficult to accept the gap between creators and users of knowledge. Those who treat patients holisticly want practical information that enhances quality care.

With new insights into social emotions, providers may begin

to see emotions, the affective components of which may even be unconscious, as a predictable element of health and illness. Emotions propel healthy people; in illness emotions become sluggish, even to the point of hindering constructive behavior. Whenever this kind of knowledge about emotions is integrated into the practice of health care, quality care should improve, but not without a price. Since primary health care involves face-to-face contact with distressed patients, quality patient care becomes quite exhausting. If there is any profession with the potential for emotional overload, it is surely health care. Fortunately, information therapy works for the provider as well as for the recipient.

Not all quality health care depends upon an individual's technical knowledge. Much of it emerges within a professional community of others—seasoned professionals to young professionals, professionals to patient, and professionals to clients. Working within these social relationships, we describe events, solve problems, develop skills, plan our careers, cope with life, and achieve remarkable successes. Whether as professionals or patients, we depend upon our acquaintances. Stressful human contact affects emotional health in much the same way that constricted coronary arteries lead to painful heart attacks.

Health providers use behavioral treatment strategies that come from such disciplines as sociology, nursing, mental health, clinical psychology, and psychiatry. Some say that diagnosing the patient's distress can be as complicated as examining the heart, where a cardiologist uses either heart catheterization or electrocardiograms. Distress intervention may not include a coronary bypass or prescription of nitroglycerin, but health providers have developed their own sophisticated approaches for patient care. Counselors, nurses, social workers, or psychologists—these inform clients about disturbing emotions and corrective actions. Their knowledge, gained over the years, occasionally does need updating as new insights and social technologies develop. These professionals must stay current if their career effectiveness is not to decline.

Another important aspect of continuing health care that may suffer is that of providing emotional support. To prevent that possibility from occuring, new approaches in health care are needed.

This thinking is shared by two respected medical educators, Karl Menninger and Rudolph J. Napodano. If Menninger's assessment of health care training is correct, then this book fills a professional need. According to him, professional health care training historically reflects an individualistic bias, both in diagnosis and intervention. After twenty-five years of clinically educating medical students, Napodano agrees. He recommends that the health care curriculum combine the rigor of scientific method with the personal sensitivity that suffering patients expect and deserve. The new curriculum should include "the teaching of empathy and compassion," along with instruction in basic and clinical sciences. Specifically, Napodano advocates courses on "ethics, socioanthropology, psychology, personal belief models, communication theory and skills, and decision theory and analysis, with carefully selected exercises and activities in the theory and skills of the traditionally taught hard sciences"(1986:17).

If medical interventions do eventually include a broader perspective than that of the individual, then sociologists can certainly make a contribution. According to Menninger, this is sound reasoning: "Every clinician can cite examples in which the nature of the individual problem did not become clear until the dynamics of the larger social system did." To stimulate and develop those insights, Menninger advocates "a systematic exposure to the concepts, the theory, the structure of disciplines of knowledge other than our own."

Menninger and Napodano's proposals for the inclusion of broad social and moral issues in a medical curriculum have found other supporters in the medical community. The Panel on the General Professional Education of the Physician and College Preparation for Medicine recommended similar curriculum changes. They advocated an expansion of subject areas to include topics on social trends and patient care. Their recommendations were similar to those of Menninger and Napodano and were designed to broaden medical training to keep pace with our rapidly changing society. If implemented, these recommendations would give medical students and other health care professionals the capacity both to adapt to those changes and to provide the services that are required. As medical educators, Menninger and Napodano are supporters of these ideas for several other reasons.

Health professionals have typically practiced medicine one-on-one with a predominant focus on bodily functions. This type of individual bias evolved until Freud diverted exclusive attention from the body to the psyche. Until now, medical intervention worked well, but current social trends now point to the need for an even greater understanding of political, social, and legal factors. Even the prime movers in shaping health care institutions are changing. These prime movers are spiraling costs, new competitive delivery systems, increased occupational specialization, continued privatization, expanding deinstitutionalization, and increasing medical liability. The old system of institutional public control is giving way to a new one: community-based, privately-owned, and profit-driven. The end result is a massive restructuring of the health industry; a fact which has direct implications for the profession.

Fortunately, this does not mean that the total number of health care professionals should decrease. Quite the contrary, if statistical trends continue. Almost 7.9 million people are employed in this industry, a 90 percent growth from 1970. Of these, 1.4 million professionals work in convalescent homes and 3.1 million work in community hospitals. Accounting for almost 40 percent of the total, registered nurses make up the largest segments (Public Health Services, 1985). Projecting out to the year 2000, analysts estimate a surplus of 300,000 health care workers. Ironically, the trend of empty hospital beds (from 25 percent nationwide in 1980 to 40 percent by 1987) must be matched against the fact that 13.6 percent of all RN positions are not filled now. If these projections do continue, the shortage of nurses will reach 1.2 million by 2000. This fact, along with the growth patterns, has serious implications. Not only are institutions changing, so are the numbers and types of professionals who work in them. Another change also seems imminent: the need to bring human dimensions into the foreground of treatment. Those who study emotions—psychiatrists, psychotherapists, clinical psychologists, mental health technicians, educational therapists, psychiatric social workers, and school health educators—probably agree. Their treatment strategies emphasize the emotional states of clients.

As an educator, I am personally concerned with balancing technical training with human understanding. In our zeal for scientific knowledge, let's not neglect the full range of emotions found in human predicaments and social problems. Any professional at disasters and emergencies will bear witness to the devastating force of these tragedies. Even so, patients and victims need friends and neighbors as well as professional help. Victims may never fully solve their emotional traumas without substituting positive feelings that are socially generated for debilitating ones that rob them of their energy. That substitution process begins by examining basic assumptions, assumptions about medical models, educational curricula, and treatment strategies. Civil defense workers, Red Cross relief workers, police officers, firemen, and rescue workers are the first to witness devastation to community life. Yet many others, including the general public, need two types of information about community sentiments and emotions. First, they need to recognize emotional variations surrounding crises, and second, they need to understand the process of becoming emotion buffers for their suffering neighbors and friends.

Part I

Recognizing the Social Context of Emotions

Chapter 1

The Emotional Side of Health

Hospitalized patients are not the only ones who worry about health or their lack of it! The next time you're walking down the aisles of the grocery store, notice how many health-related items there are on the shelves, everything from Preparation H to pregnancy tests. While self diagnosis works on a simple headache, it lacks the precision and sophistication needed for the persistent migraines of the Type A person. Even the well-intentioned office worker, giving herself a pregnancy test during lunch break, can make a mistake or be mislead by "sound" advice. You don't have to read Mark Twain to find out about Aunt Polly's snake oil treatments.

Americans flocked to Mexican Laetrile Clinics not only for the cure of cancer, but also for countless "quick cures" of arthritis. After spending one month and thousands of dollars in a Tijuana clinic, a 55-year-old man with inoperative lung cancer found out too late about medical quackery south of the border. Instead of Aunt Polly, he found a doctor who was much more sympathetic than any he had found on this side of the border. Upon returning home with a three-month supply, he began taking Laetrile. Ignorant of the placebo effect from his optimism about a cure, and discounting the temporary remission from earlier radiation in an American hospital, Jack honestly believed that the battle for restored health was over—right up until his death (Anastas, 1986:86-90).

Dr. Charles Moertel, professor of oncology at the Mayo Clinic, called Laetrile "one of the major health problems of our time. The Laetrile folks were very skillful in organizing the press to present their case, and they sold the American public on Laetrile as a cancer cure." And a convincing sell it was: 1) Harris recorded a 30 percent margin for legalization, 2) twenty-seven states passed the laws, 3) people trusted their instincts over standard medical testing, and 4) an Oklahoma federal court ruled it legal with some restrictions. The Food and Drug Administration rejected it, however, and a federal appeals court overturned the earlier Oklahoma federal court ruling (O'Hara,1987).

Arthritis cases may not be as dramatic as cancer, but they also represent the quest for wholeness. Thousands of arthritis sufferers drink healing water, sit hours steaming in mineral baths, endure all kinds of diets, put medicinal mud on the affected areas, and even wear copper bracelets (Anastas, 1986:86-90). Television commercials and magazine ads that push youth and beauty are everywhere in our culture, but these say less about the power of marketing than about the intense longing for wholeness.

Everyone wants health and wholeness, but everyone does not agree on the treatments for illness, injury, and old age because evaluation standards differ. On the one hand, medical professionals use sophisticated high-tech instruments which can detect the slightest deviation from normal. This modern technology gives facts, not conjectures, about medical problems. On the other hand, the sick person depends upon intuition—based on feelings and fears—to interpret bodily variations from one moment to the next. Unfortunately, many patients trust the opinions of their neighbor down the street more than they do those of the doctor in the clinic. Suzanne White, an historian and archivist with the Food and Drug Administration, equates this simple trust to lack of comprehension: "When medicine is beyond the reach of the common man in terms of understanding, he tends to trust his own wits."

How do we interpret this strange mixture of emotions, intentions, judgments, and actions? We do know that people want compassionate care. Porter Memorial Hospital in Denver conducted a three-year study to determine what people look for in health care. Richard D. Stier, vice president for marketing, found that people want: 1) information about their condition, 2) attention to patients and their families, and 3) good nursing care. These top three items involve the human touch. The other rankings are more impersonal: medical equipment, reputation, price, specialists, efficient procedures, visiting hours, location, parking, and comfortable rooms.

People don't understand medical procedures, but they do understand quality care. The challenge is to make scientific, high-tech procedures and medicine more palatable to the patient. Professionals who maintain trust levels and communicate may also attract more patients than those who do not. Their patients have the benefits of both quality relations and scientific treatment.

Let's consider eight pertinent questions about this emotional side of health: What? Where? How? Why? Who? When? So What? and Now What? Obviously, emotions figure into the equation of people's desire for healthy lives. That basic observation has important implications for health providers. As we explore these eight questions about emotional health, we will find some answers to the ambivilance of human nature.

Encapsulated Emotions

What do intense, sometimes misguided, concerns for health mean for the provider? That is the first of our eight questions. Encapsulated emotions are confusing to the average patient, but not to the health care professionals who regularly see these emotions. Four types of patients reveal their complexity: 1) When the healthy are feeling sick, they experience more and more the depths of encapsulated emotions that lie dormant within them; 2) When the sick are feeling healthy, they experience the depths of depression less and less; 3) Moderately sick people are aware that they are not well; 4) completely well people don't believe that they are sick. We all appreciate something, or someone, the most after we've lost it. We realize its true value, as in the case of health, only after it's taken from us. It is after the loss that we feel the depths of our encapsulated emotions. So "hardly-ever-been-well" sick people appreciate being well and respect illness; "never-been-sick" well people don't do either.

If there were only some way to channel this emotional concern for one's health into a proper treatment modality based on scientific fact, then health care would be not only a true partnership but also a joint venture for improving public health statistics. What's the solution? It's not possible to completely educate every citizen about all facets of health care; nor can every sick person be hospitalized to ensure proper diagnosis and treatment. Even if individual patients could understand their medical problem, that does not guarantee that they would be able to treat themselves. And for each seriously ill patient admitted to a hospital and successfully recovering against all odds, there may be dozens who are not. Both ingredients are desirable: emotional concern for one's health and scientific application to ensure the best treatment.

That standard (encapsulated emotional concerns and professional judgment) becomes the benchmark for recognizing any and all medical problems of the patient. But if and when both ingredients are not present, no one is satisfied. Then both provider and recipient realize the importance of total health care. Emotionally discouraged patients are much harder to care for, compared to those making rapid progress. Ironically, they are the ones who need emotional support the most. Health professionals often marvel at the difference that emotional encouragement and support can make. If only positive emotions, like so many pints of blood, could be stored (encapsulated) for an emergency and then injected into the discouraged and anxious patient as needed. The closest remedies for this dilemma that we have are the various psychotropic medications. The most prescribed medications in our society today are the anxiolytic drugs known as librium, valium, and ativan, which not only relax muscles, but also reduce anxiety.

Although mind-altering drugs effectively sedate the anxious patient, they are no substitute for either emotional support from outside or the emotional capacities found within. The long-term effects of encapsulated emotions, while often not a substitute for some medication, may actually increase the likelihood of recovery and continued stability. Health care includes not only the art of medicine, but also the science of understanding. Since even a partial emotional paralysis is a fearful and mysterious obstacle to a patient's recovery, even a small amount of emotional support might make the difference in getting the patient "back on their feet."

Now for the second of our eight questions: Where are emotions located? Is it possible for providers to know precisely where emotions come from? Beyond physical problems, what else happens to patients before and after major surgery? We may not be able to X-ray emotions as easily as bones, but we can easily locate four types of emotions in patients. Of four strata where emotions are located, "sensible feelings" is the first one and the most visibly felt and known. Intense pain overloads bodily sensations and tends to obliterate all other levels of emotion (Denzin, 1984:118-120).

The second stratum of emotions is described as "intentional value feelings" (Denzin,1984:120-125). These emotions push patients away from their isolated bodily experience and pull them toward meaningful associations with others. What begins in the body as sense awareness merges into this second emotional strata. Denzin makes a distinction between bodily felt and mentally expressed emotions. Patients identify their moods through this capacity. Depending upon current circumstances, patients use these expressions of feelings such as "sorrowful," "depressed," "exhausted," or "wearisome."

In the first emotional stratum, patients sense painful stimuli; in the second stratum, they share that "lived feeling" socially with others. This distinction between individually felt physical pain (first stratum) and socially shared feelings (second stratum) has import for providers. The bodily pain of grief is individually felt by those affected; however, feelings about that grief can be collectively shared. It is through the "feelings of the lived body" (the second stratum) that patients share how they feel in their present physical state.

The third stratum consists of "feelings of the self and the moral person." This stratum extends emotions even further from the self (Denzin,1984:120-125). After a painful surgery, a patient recognizes pain (level one) and describes it (level two) to providers. Next, the patient (level three) assigns a value to what happened and discusses these values objectively. Surgery is personal, yet it is objectively evaluated by an ideal standard. Emotions in this stratum don't connect with sensible or lived body feelings. They are outside the body but inside the value system of the community. Patients use such terms as "exhaustion," "fatigue," "exhilaration," and "satiation" (Denzin,1984:127).

The fourth stratum of emotions deals with "feelings of self worth." It connects the provider and patient as people. People form a community "not conditioned by external value complexes," but by common feelings of worth, dignity, and respect. Denzin uses the phrase "moral worth," and identifies these emotions by such terms as "ashamed," "disgusted," or "defeated." Easy to identify, but difficult to understand, these emotions are tied directly to the patient's sense of worth. Standards of worth emerge from a culture, but individuals use them to evaluate their own worth. What is outside the person is internalized, so self-worth is evaluated independently of any immediate crisis. Consequently, this emotional stratum gives patients an identity greater than themselves. From this stratum come worth, meaning, and purpose for life itself (Denzin,1984:125).

These four strata of emotions allow patients to transcend their problems either individually or collectively. They connect the provider with the patient in a complex array of emotional patterns. The higher forms of emotions allow the providers to identify with patients, even beyond their immediate feelings. Intense feelings are shared even beyond the first stratum of emotions. Though often invisible, emotions, like diseases, are infectious, identifiable, and communicable. These patterns of expressing emotions form the basis for understanding one another within the health community and communicating meaningfully at deeper levels. This is why health care is a personal transaction.

Perplexities of Illness

While hospitalized patients aren't the only ones who agonize over their lack of wholeness, they are the ones best aided by both combinations of the health standards that we discussed at the beginning of this chapter—their own intuitive feelings and the medical facts. Surprisingly, these two standards sometimes do converge and become visible enough for providers to realize how (question three) they can respond to others.

Smith (1981) interviewed eighty-six patients recovering from acute or severe illnesses. These interviews also revealed the same four levels of emotions. Since level one is specific (body sensations, pain, and discomfort), only the others wil be discussed here. Stratum two (lived feelings or feelings about feelings) is identified in Smith's interviews by predictable quotes reflecting depression, exhaustion, and weariness: "This comes as a real setback." "I'm trapped." "I'm so depressed." While these feelings come from within, they also move outward, affecting others. One patient said of time management: "Now I realize I have to take time for myself, and I want more time and energy with my family, especially my children."

Intentional values, the third stratum, are attributed to subjective feelings. While personal,these feelings fit into an interpretive framework which gives collective meaning to pain or suffering (Denzin,1984:120-121). These feelings form the basis for interacting with empathizers, including sensitive health professionals: "The staff seem to manage to have time whenever anyone is upset. They never talk down to us or act as though we're no good. That means so much." " Nobody here treats us like dirt. Nobody puts us down." In other words, objective meaning is attached to the patients' suffering through interaction with medical staff.

Finally, there is the fourth type of emotion—those positive, yet difficult expressions about lessons learned. They are identified by words of self-worth or worthlessness: "disgusted,"or "defeated."

Once expressed, these emotions are easily identified. However, such admissions aren't easy to make, and some patients may be reluctant to reveal such feelings. Nevertheless, patients often describe those difficulties in terms of personal growth: "It's as though I've suddenly grown up and become aware of a whole side of life I never knew was there." "I never used to be aware of people around me—how they might feel or what they might be going through." According to Denzin, this emotion connects feelings about self and the moral person together. This emotion also includes feelings about one's self (shame, disgust, pride, self-defeat), character, spirit, or presence. It is not surprising that Smith recorded examples of people experiencing a spiritual renewal: "Illness has crystallized my faith." Through interviews with 115 others surviving tragedies, Veninga (1985:217) also identified this fourth emotional type: "I think that without God I probably would have had a mental breakdown....I believed that God knew who I was and why I was so angry and accepted me for who I am. That belief—that I could be myself—was healing"(1985:217). "I can't explain it, but I went into that chapel crushed. And I came out feeling strong"(1985:218).

Obviously, these emotional struggles extend beyond the major physical problems. Feelings also come from less acute illness and are regularly shared with professionals in routine health care procedures. Any illness requires positive reinforcement if people are to maximize their chances of recovery (Smith,1981). This support includes appraisal, information, affirmation, and emotional support (Brown, 1986:4-9). However severe the illness or surgery, once the recovery begins, patients cue their own monitoring system. The character of these cues was identified through two-hundred patients who freely expressed their readiness for discharge (Smith 1981). To identify the diversity of responses (feeling cues), the researcher used five categories:

1) Increased strength and energy (physical cues)

2) The ability to care for oneself (capacity cues)
3) A desire to return to normal (feeling tone cues)
4) A physician's decision (external cues)
5) Support from family or friends (external cues)

When asked about their readiness to leave, patients discussed these cues and their perceived significance for recovery. Item three, the feeling cues, linked physical abilities (sensible feelings) with the providers or supporters (lived feelings). Patients estimated their readiness for leaving the hospital through conversations with physicians, friends, and family. Even though the physician makes the final release decision, most patients made their own evaluation of their physical condition and estimated their capacity to resume their former responsibilities.

Their accuracy does not always follow the actual diagnosis, but the fact remains that people do monitor their physical and emotional conditions throughout an illness. Accuracy did depend, however, upon certain social factors: economic status, religion, sex, age, and type of treatment. These factors define the social context where definitions of situations begin. It is not surprising that high measures of socio-economic status and religiosity correlate with a high degree of accuracy in self appraisal. Middle class professionals accurately describe their own capacities, feelings, and physical conditions. In contrast, Hispanic patients depend more on family and friends in making predictions about recovery. Women openly express their emotions more than men. Predictably, the elderly need more reassurance, and psychiatric patients registered less family support. Question four of our eight questions asks why emotional health works this way?

Health Care as Transactions

Why are emotions important? Why is health care a social transaction? To answer these questions is to explain why patients seek stabilizing emotions from others in times of crisis. Emotions are an important dimension of health care; there is a connection between illness, a patient's assessments of it, and the emotional feelings that follow. In a care-giving situation, one person (the patient) meaningfully interacts with another (the provider) or a group (family and friends). This in turn results in emotional bonding at the deepest levels. To be sure, specifics make a difference in how much is communicated. Nevertheless, patients who disclose their true feelings become, paradoxically, more vulnerable. That has both negative and positive consequences; people's pains are painful, and pain brings intense struggles. From these encounters come greater understanding about, and frustrations with, emotions normally reserved for the very closest of family or friends. Emotions give us understanding beyond the factual level; a person enters into another's world of meaning. We use descriptive terms such as "sympathy," "empathy," "sympathetic understanding," "introspection," and "verstehen" (Denzin,1984:131-133). All of which suggest that health care is transactional.

Not everyone responds in the same way to crisis, illness, or surgery. Nor does that emotional response stay constant, as any provider of health care knows. Regardless of the patient's response, health care is a social transaction in which providers create a climate where either positive or dissogenic feelings flourish. This can clearly be seen in the case of children. When a hospitalized seven-year-old "plays nurse" with her Raggedy Ann doll, she eases her fears about surgery and nurses. It creates a positive atmosphere where she learns not only about her surgery, but also about her anxieties. These procedures vary with age and length of stay. Relaxed by board games, older children tend to reveal their true feelings. These and other approaches help to release excessive emotional energy. In each case the climate depends upon the medical staff. "Utilizing laughter during nursing care and play with pediatric patients decreases tension and promotes pleasurable feelings in both the child and the nurse" (D'Antonio, 1984:358). The point is that play promotes informality, and patients share "in a non-threatening way the full range of emotions" (Jack, 1987:17).

Sharing is cathartic, relieving the tensions of those playing. In fact, "people who include play in their lifestyle may be healthier physically, and better able to handle the stresses of daily demands" (Jack, 1987:20).

Everyone responds differently to crisis, illness, or surgery. All emotions are not negative. Emotions fluctuate, but why? The explanation comes from the creative provider who analyzes the case. Normally, these explanations—found in the biomedical models of disease—account for biological differences. This particular model predisposes health care providers to conceptualize diseases and therapies as discreetly isolated entities. This cause and effect analysis is consistent not only with the biological and physical sciences, but also with biomedicine as an extension of these basic sciences.

Providers exclusively trained to deal with biological phenomena may also need models which are more applicable to higher levels of interaction involving more complex behavior patterns. Experimentally, placebos often produce rather dramatic differences in a patient's condition, not to mention the positive interaction between people. Why should scientists measure these positive social transactions? Cousins says that they should because positive emotions explain why some terminally ill patients defy their poor prognosis for survival and live beyond what is normally expected. Without emotional support, only half of the patient is being treated, for "emotional needs are as great as the physical needs" (Cousins, 1985:96). Is there medical evidence that positive transactions have any physiological effect? Cousins thinks so, and cites as evidence the medical research of Walter Cannon, who found that heightened emotional states can increase the number of red blood cells 10 to 15 percent. Health care providers who believe that "hope and confidence and faith are as much a part of a strategy for recovery as anything" (Cousins, 1985:97) should therefore encourage their patients whenever possible.

Many care givers intuitively interact with their patients on higher levels. Professionals may also deliberately approach illness and treatment in an integrated fashion—combining the biological and behavioral aspects of illness. This is social realism, because most patients already interact with themselves, health professionals, family members, and friends as they seek gains from their losses. Such transactions highlight not only disruption, but also social reconstruction.

The sociology of emotions supplements what is neglected in the biomedical model. "The social scientist's preference for the strictly scientific posture, at the possible expense of clinical relevance, is not altogether surprising..." (Bloch and Crouch, 1985:244). For an analysis on the emotional side of health to be clinically relevant, it should begin where the three interacting parties—patient, provider, and supporter—also begin in health care. Engel (1980) develops a biopsychosocial model not only for analytical purposes, but also for clinical applications. His systems hierarchy begins at the level of atoms and molecules and moves toward the personal experiences of people in families, communities, and nations.

One issue of this model is how the hierarchy of levels interfaces, for that in turn affects how much attention a particular level gets. Some therapists are purists who are limited to one and only one technique; others are integralists using a variety of techniques. The purists represent the traditional approach, while the second group represents the eclectic approach. Eclecticism is prominent in "the Palo Alto MRI (Mental Research Institute) models, integrative problem-centered therapy..., integrative multi-level therapy..., and the psychoeducational family models" (Sugarman,1986:3). These clinicians merge various levels based on the realism of social interaction. To eliminate confusion over particular combinations, Sugarman gives four guidelines. He believes that an approach should be: 1) consistent with the therapeutic goals, 2) justifiably chosen, 3) appropriate to the patient, and 4) synergistically enhancing (Sugarman, 1986:10). Engle's model of higher emotional levels and systems hiararchy raises questions about providing health care through intensive social interaction.

Intensive Social Interaction

Engle's biopsychosocial model is perhaps too complex. A more appropriate question is this: Who (question five of our eight) is involved in providing health care? Such a model is found in the Intensive Social Interaction model shown in Figure 1-1.

This greatly simplified model shows the significant interaction between and among the patient, the provider, and the supporters. Napodano's teaching philosophy, consistent with the Intensive Social Interaction (ISI) model, assumes a particular strategy for

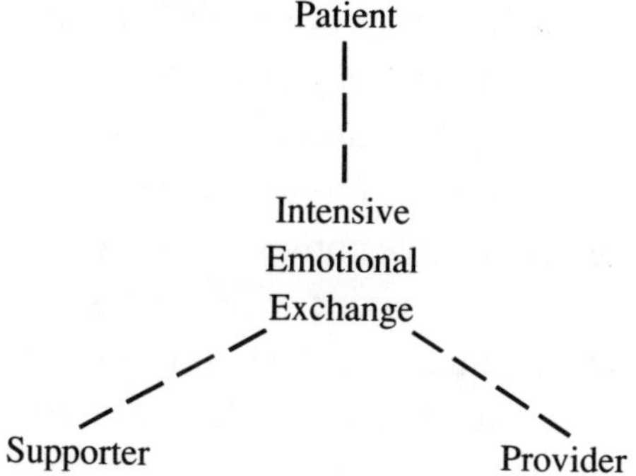

Figure 1-1. Intensive Social Interaction.

teaching medical practice. His philosophy also stresses the important interaction between the patient and physician. As a scientist involved in healing, Napodano emphasizes the teaching of empathy and compassion along with biotechnology and basic science. Napodano advocates five objectives for medical practice:

1) To be clinically competent
2) To be patient-centered
3) To care for patients as well as cure them
4) To have a decision-making perspective
5) To work toward a synthesis

Health care professionals must first be competent, but Napodano recommends a patient-focused orientation. This means that the patient and his specific needs are given top priority. What is required of providers in giving top priority to specific patient problems? Napodano lists helping attitudes and behavior as the qualitative dimension. That means that the "concept of altruistic 'care' ought to be added to the notion of 'cure' " (1986:96). Yet this qualitative and humanitarian factor comes only as a professional becomes "a human who also experiences feelings and frustrations when things do not go well" (1986:99). It is that potential human quality from which compassion, sympathy, and empathy flow—emotions which we will discuss at length in Chapter 2.

To accomplish his first three objectives for medical practice, we must also have Napodano's fourth and fifth components: a decision-making perspective and some type of synthesis. The basis for a decision-making perspective comes from combining the following: facts with attitudes, behavior with beliefs, clinical medicine with cultural practices, quality care with technical skill, and adequate diagnosis with mutual consent. Here is how he expresses the fifth objective of teaching the healing sciences: "I have heard many physicians state that the psychosocial, cultural, ethical, and belief-system issues that relate to an illness are not a part of the physician's job. They belong to the nurse, the social worker, the clergy. I do not agree. The physician ought always to remain the central person in the care of the patient" (1986:113). Socializing the young professional in the proper care of the sick is an important part of the training.

The ISI Model links not only the provider to the patient, but the supporters as well. Without supporters, a patient must cope with these stress levels alone. Smaller family units and declining social support exacerbate the problem. Only friendless people really need supporters; only friendly people have them. The worse off a patient is, the more friends are needed, yet the less they are available. This problem is compounded as more people are placed under health care supervision for longer periods of time. Medical science not only gives longer life, but requires more intensive health care. Only supporters truly give emotional, material, informational, and appraisal support. *The patient finds relief most when social supporters help buffer the emotional trauma of critical events* (Brown, 1986:4-9). Research shows that patient anxiety, a "transitory emotional state of tension and apprehension," varies inversely with the climate of interpersonal relationships. This is also true not only for the patient's emotional health, but also for others forming this ISI network (Bramwell and Whall, 1986).

Hardiness and Health

Now for the sixth question: When are people the most healthy? If the standard is health and wholeness, it might make sense to reverse the line of questioning. Rather than ask what makes people sick, health care professionals should also ask how the healthy stay well. By reversing the question, we could then cover the full range from wholeness to sickness.

Stressful life events aggravate or provoke illness (Holmes and Rahe,1967; Dohrewend and Dohrewend,1974). These researchers measured those events which produce the greatest stress, it is not surprising that they ignored the psychosocial factors which might moderate stress. These factors need attention, particularly in our discussion of emotional health. Information about factors which buffer the individual from stress can be found in research studies on the hardy personality.

Some individuals remain healthy despite stressful events: job transfer, death, divorce, marriage, illness. Individual characteristics and coping strategies determine when people are the most healthy. These factors have been the goal of researchers in their search for the answer to this question of "When?" Though the research objects vary, the basic assumption does not: some people have an existential orientation to life which gives them an advantage (Kobasa,1982:6). Existentialists see life as "being-in-process," a take charge activity; it demands something from us. This attitude may contribute to their healthiness.

After conducting extensive research on executives under stress, Kobasa (1979) found that some executives coped better with negative events and circumstances than others. Those most able to cope were identified as hardy personalities. According to Kobasa, this type of individual is not stable by inactivity; rather, they are hardy by their dynamic, active life style. By means of a certain life style, these hardy individuals reduce much of the negative effects of a stressful environment. They exhibit three characteristics: commitment, control, and challenge.

Let's take them in that order and discuss each individually. Commitment entails the belief, confidence, and ability that one can manage one's life, even under stressful circumstances. This means that hardy individuals have a greater capacity to adjust and still achieve their life goals. One major finding is of particular relevance to our study of social emotions: the importance of commitment "more than self-esteem or personal competence, because it is based in a sense of community" (Kobasa,1982:7). Being involved with other people is the most important characteristic.

The second characteristic of the hardy personality is control, the inner strength and determination toward action that seems to minimize some of the stress. This develops as the person balances his sense of purpose with a commitment to activities. People want to know "why" things happen the way they do. Their desire to know leads them to explore other options. Finally, Kobasa found that the notion of challenge was important to hardy people. Hardy individuals have the capacity to see beyond the problem and somehow accept stressful events as challenges in life, enabling them to respond constructively to difficulties. This means that such people believe in change as a norm of life; therefore, they take risks. But they also consolidate available resources when faced with stressful events.

Studying the hardiness and mental health of immigrants, Kuo and Yung-Mei found some significant correlations. Those immigrants who exhibited ruggedness, assertiveness, and self determination experienced less depression. The researchers concluded that the hardy personality averted much of the stress "associated with migration" (1986:147). In other words, the loss of a secure environment is mitigated by a hardy personality and social relationships. Like Kobasa, these two researchers also found *a sense of community to be very important as an emotional insulator during difficult times*. Obviously, these are not the only factors associated with healthy individuals. There are other factors revealed by medical histories, such as hereditary and genetic factors, and constitutional predispositions. An individual thus instinctively and biologically responds to crisis. Even allowing for these biological factors, it is evident that different life styles and behavioral approaches do affect the response to emotional crises.

When are health professionals the most likely to endure stressful activities? What does research show about their ability to overcome a stressful environment? Surprisingly, hardy nurses in surgical and medical ICUs in a university hospital experienced no higher levels of burnout than others in nonstressful hospital environments. The important factor of hardiness—buffering the high levels of stress— was evident in all units of the hospital. By comparing the hardy and nonhardy nurses, the researchers noted that hardiness made the difference. Those nurses who demonstrated high professional commitment, maintained personal control, and accepted the challenges of the job also experienced lower stress. Above all, "lack of control over negative events" was shown to correlate highest with stress levels and the burnout syndrome (Keane, et al., 1985). This fact is especially relevant in recent discussions about Type A behavior. It now appears that the principle emotional factors accounting for coronary risk are hostility, anger, and mistrust (Matthews and Haynes, 1986).

Sickness and Disease

Granting the importance of hardiness, so what now? This is our seventh question—So what? We can define preventive medicine as seeing the whole person before and after an illness, wondering about social conditions which promote sickness, closely analyzing the public health statistics, and analyzing personal behavior and life styles. Is this the purpose of health care? Is this the cause to which professionals are to be committed? It is ironic, but apparently so (based on public health statistics), that affluence in money, food, and leisure can actually lead to unhealthy conditions. As a by-product of life in an affluent society, many people don't protect their health. They eat excessively, fail to exercise regularly, and live hurried lives with little time for rest. All of these factors are directly related to mortality. Unhealthy life style plays a significant role in many of the most common fatal illnesses in this country. One of the major causes of death is lung cancer (92,000 men and 44,000 women died of it in 1988). An estimated 320,000 more will die from smoking-related diseases. All of these deaths could be avoided by a change in life style that eliminated the smoking habit.

One wonders how long more monies can be put into health care programs. Already the amount has increased from $27 billion (1960) to $287 billion (1981); Stanhope and Lancaster (1984:ix) question whether these resources are spent wisely: "Health care monies have largely been allocated to the treatment of disease rather than to prevention. In an era of economic constraints, how long will it be feasible to support a 'fix-it' orientation to health care?"

The absence of physical illness does not necessarily mean a person is well. To be healthy, from a sociological perspective, implies that people reach their potential in all areas of social life: physical, emotional, and social. The inability to function at every level of social life suggests some type of disease. Thus, health implies more than just biological fitness. We can also ask who is responsible for the unhealthy conditions which ultimately lead to sickness and disease. The answer to that question involves either the health care system or the individual, or both. We might initially suppose that an approach involving both the individual and the system would be the best course of action. But is it? "The health care system typically becomes activated when an illness is detected" (Lancaster and Lancaster, 1984:33). The issues raised by such a discussion are illustrated in Table 1-1.

Table 1-1. Expanding Health Matters

Location	Orientation	Focus	Example	Model
Medical Clinic	Physical Disease	Entity	Polio	Biological
Emergency Room	Social Stress	Dignity	Abuse	Behavioral

If health concerns expand beyond the medical clinic, shouldn't health care? How might this happen? Health teams may medically do what they can for the sick, but there remain certain illnesses, or aspects thereof, which no amount of medicine can cure. Is there any reason to suppose that alternative interventions might effectively supplement raditional medical treatments? A patient who is not given some dignity or respect by a partner probably won't recover from the resulting emotional deficiency even in a hospital emergency room. Abuse in any number of forms contributes to social stress. Just as polio once brought people to seek medical help, spouse abuse now brings them to the emergency room. No physical problem is isolated. Medical staff must interact with these people and recognize the social implications. Life may have always been stressful, but only recently have we begun to monitor these social problems.

Basic Assumptions, Conclusions

Now what does all of this mean (the eighth and last of our questions on emotional health)? One of the major requirements of health professionals (counselors, nurses, social workers, psychologists, physicians) is to inform their clients, utilizing the information gained from their professional training and education. Such insights, when applied in a specific social environment, can be used to develop healthier life styles. The orientation for counselors and clients is in the applied sciences, whatever the specific disease or crisis. *In other words, the nexus for both the health professional and the patient is the search for information which, when applied, helps to prevent further emotional distress, mental anguish, or physical complications.* This point of contact with others represents a social pattern vital to recovery. It is also the sensitive nexus of interaction which forms the basis for the following assumptions:

1) People's emotions are socially based.
2) Emotions are basic to mental health.
3) Emotions occur at three levels of experience.
4) Life styles affect emotional health.
5) Intervention skills can be learned.
6) These skills work best with sociological interpretations.

There are implications for these assumptions—practical steps to take in analyzing and prescribing intervention strategies. There is a logical rationale for making these assumptions. In order to assist others in coping with stress, the following steps should be covered.

1) An awareness of what's emotionally happening to the individual.
2) The ability to step back and see oneself sociologically.
3) Corrective measures which will ensure emotional stability.

Towards this end, then, this book is directed: that health professionals will supplement their training with sociological insights Such insights provide a sense of professional competence, as well as the specific skills necessary to cope effectively and efficiently with patients/clients. Once this happens, we can all learn how to step back, empathize, and incorporate our training to guide others.

Since health care is a stressful profession, this book can be used not only to gain insights about the emotions of illness, but also to provide valuable information about the personal stress of the health care professional. If patients experience high levels of emotional stress, then surely those providing health care will also be affected. Maslanch (1979:114-119) verified this assumption and explored ways for health care professionals to cope with the problem of burnout. He listed a number of helpful coping behaviors for the professional: learning more about emotional elements; understanding distressing experiences; gaining support from associates; using humor as a release; separating work and play; and maintaining good physical health. *All of these strategies buffer health professionals from excessive stress.* More so than with other professions, the health care profession involves intense social interaction and excessive emotional stress.

Providers can gain social insights into important health care topics, but this means applying a sociological analysis to the health profession. The social dimensions are already there, but not highlighted as in this text. Traditionally, sociologists don't ask the eight questions listed above. Rather, they question how social patterns affect health and disease and how the patient's values, attitudes, and life style determine what action is taken. Yet what should be explored is *the emotional side of health care*: how people cope with disrupted social relations; exactly how people buffer emotions; and what resources increase their capacity to cope effectively with them. There is much that we don't know about emotions, but some aspects of emotions seem obvious: every patient has them; some can be positive, although most are not; emotions are handled in a social context both in and out of the hospital; and finally, emotions are an integral part of who we are—not a fragmented piece of how we feel.

This book has one thesis: *patients should freely express their emotions as naturally as they express their physical ailments.* Both of these freedoms increase their capacity to control otherwise uncontrolled emotions. This increased capacity should thereby accelerate emotional and physical healing. But much of this healing depends upon those most directly involved with patients during the health crisis. For this reason, ideas about the social dynamics of emotions should be closely connected to health care.

Chapter 2

Tracking Emotions in Self and Society

Other than the Karolinska Institute in Stockholm, only Los Angeles has a Center for Preventive Psychiatry. In August 1987, UCLA established this Center for the purpose of detecting and preventing emotional disorders. While heralded as an innovation, the Center follows a time-honored tradition of tracking emotions in self and society (Simross, 1987).

The extent of this American tradition is measured by two University of Michigan surveys (Adelmann, 1987). In 1957, and again in 1976, researchers discovered that an ever increasing number of Americans sought emotional counseling (14 percent versus 26 percent). By comparing these two bench marks, researchers made several other discoveries. They learned that the Freudian tradition peaked by 1957; that affluence and transportation influenced life more than church or community; that ordinary people sought advice; that problems—illness, death, parenting—prompted people to seek help; that people worried more about personal fulfillment than maladjustment.

The drama of emotions in self and society continues to change. Just as changing weather brings an uncontrollable cough or sneeze, so these social changes bring unhealthy emotions. People today seek out others, less as a platform to express their views, and more as a community to share their feelings. Even so, about 20 percent of us experience severe emotional drainage and need qualified professionals to provide assistance. That assistance comes from paraprofessionals, self-help groups, and families who share personal problems and the desire for self improvement. Understanding how emotions develop in self and society is a modern quest. To visualize self is to see an emerging, passionate entity full of sentiments. Never were these passions explored more systematically than by Freud at the turn of the century. His ideas about personality continue to influence the health professions, as do Jung's ideas on social sentiments. Rather than isolate the self, Jung viewed it in a sociohistorical context. This is the subject of this chapter: tracking modern ideas about human emotions by looking at the passions of self and the sentiments of society.

Because major life events register our emotions, our attempts to recall or forget what happened once again prompts emotions. Our earliest images are reservoirs of feelings. Sometimes we helplessly tolerate, rather than deliberately release, our negative reactions. This process can be seen when we are confronted with such pronouncements as: "you're diabetic," or "you have AIDS," or "we diagnosed your case as incurable cancer." Such negative information precipitates everything from shock and anger to depression and anxiety. That restricted origin of—yet broad release from—stimulated emotions continues to fascinate the public and professional alike.

A close look at health and self reveals some surprises about emotions. The word "health" comes from the Anglo-Saxon word "hail" or the later term "hol." Both words conveyed a greeting of wholeness. "Hale" meant "physical well-being be with you." Thus the word "health" suggests that our well-being depends upon the initial and subsequent greetings of others. If the greetings contain good will, then health follows. Otherwise, both good will and physical well-being are absent.

Both clinicians and practitioners discovered a similar connection between emotional health and social interaction. To track emotions in self and society, we will classify emotions into types—neurotic or normal. The former classification is associated with the Freudian view of emotions; the latter is more social or environmental in nature. Although these two traditions emerged quite differently, they do have similar features. Both are concerned with the relationship between self and society, with the Freudian view slanted toward the individual, and the latter view emphasizing the social context. Both traditions explained how emotions manifest themselves in vicious outbreaks as well as normal development. Both were concerned with health: what prevents healthy emotions and what prevails in healthy emotions. This convergence continues to capture the attention of clinicians and social scientists.

Neurotic Behavior and Emotions

It is not unusual for clinicians to differ over interpretations of emotions. Freud and Jung's divergent views are worth knowing. Theirs was the time and the place where modern interpretations of emotions began. If either is true, then there are definite reasons to explore their disagreements and their writings. Let us, therefore, try to understand why they parted company and what it means for us today.

Patients sometimes experience emotional distress over their treatment and need additional care. These feelings are not dependent upon unsuccessful treatment. Even if the surgeon successfully removes the woman's breast cancer, this does not necessarily mean the end of health care. Such successes may not address the emotions of the patient.

The early writings of Freud and Jung contain profound insights into the emotional side of health care. Sigmund Freud was the founder of psychoanalysis, and Carl Jung was his most devoted disciple. An overview of their work and an understanding of why they parted company can give us some valuable insights into the issues surrounding the concept of quality health care today.

It is possible to isolate the specific issues of disagreement between Freud and Jung. Their disagreement springs from a fundamental distinction about human nature and emotions. According to Freud's interpretation, his patients displayed emotional outbursts because they were by nature emotional creatures. Freud saw emotions as basically biological urges that originate deep within the human being. He connected these urges with the primordial period and earliest development of the race. From time to time these urges spring forth uncontrollably; typical of children when they display their displeasure as fits of passion. More visible in infancy, these urges dominate most of the child's actions because the superego (moral restraints) is less developed. With the socialization and internalization of social morality, these urges lose some of their control over the person. In time, social values are infused into the superego, giving it more control. Until this point, however, the id is free to exploit its habitat in a narcisstic and self-centered way.

In a study sponsored by the Illinois Children and Family Services Department, many teenage mothers described early experiences not too different from those of Freud's patients (Schultz,1987). Sixty percent of these teens were sexually abused, some as young as two, many under 12. All were emotionally damaged and confused about sex. Ironically, these same teens as mothers don't seem able to protect their babies from the same fate. So the cycle continues.

Even though a pregnant teenager may desperately want unconditional love, in contrast to the sexual abuse she's experienced; and even though she honestly believes that her unborn baby can fulfill her emotional need for acceptance and affection; those intense beliefs and feelings don't match reality. No one can realistically expect a newborn—incapable of returning love—to fill such an emotional void.

Freud located these types of animal behavior, instincts, and passions deep within the person's inner unconsciousness. Because these inner forces were unknown, he first used dream analysis as a means of reaching them. Through psychoanalytic sessions and reflective observations of his own childhood experience, Freud became increasingly convinced that adult dreams are really infantile sex wishes in disguise. He tried to uncover and interpret these biological drives in his patients. Today psychoanalysts assist emotionally distressed people by locating the source of their anxieties. This comes about through insights that often stem from early relationships with parents.

What is the source of anxiety? In contrast to psychodynamic therapy, rational therapists take a different approach by guiding their clients as they eliminate these irrational, destructive patterns. On the other hand, behaviorists hope to reshape behavior through rewards and punishment, a strategy of relearning. Just as many modern therapists disagree with Freud. So did Jung. It was Freud's interpretation of anxiety that ultimately contributed to the rapid decline and final termination of their relationship.

Jung, like systems therapists of today, believed that experiences within the social context produce anxiety. Jung did not believe in "half-tamed demons that inhabit the human beast." Emotions may be explosively unpredictable and even damaging, but why exaggerate emotions as Freud did by saying that clinicians who "wrestle with them" are not left "unscathed" by their viciousness. That explanation was too confusing and narrow for Jung's liking.

In a positive sense, Jung saw emotions as the source of movement from "darkness into light." Never do we realize that more than when we're least able to produce emotions. In times of crisis or distress, emotional transformations—not analytical explanations—are the best medicine. Without emotions, however, that transformation cannot begin. Such a conclusion follows from Jung's basic assumption—that emotions provide the energy for our fantasies. Emotions motivate us in our life's journeys. Freud generally emphasized the body—its unconscious influence on the psyche—while Jung viewed the interrelationships between unconscious and psyche in a much broader scope so that they took on a "universal and transcendental reality" (Morgan, 1986:223). Some have questioned the scientific validity of such a view, but Jung's idea of the "collective unconscious" is not too different from Durkheim's concept of collective consciousness. Both concepts recognize social facts which are not visible, which transcend time and space, and which influence community life. These ideas are akin to Einstein's when he "dematerialized our understanding of the physical world" (1986:223). In fact, it has been argued by Morgan that

Einstein's concept of physical energy parallels Jung's notion of psyche energy, which should not surprise us too much since Jung and Einstein were friends (1986:223).

Another similarity can be drawn from the writings of Max Weber and his concept of bureaucracy. According to Weber, if the purest form of organization exists, then the aspects of human encounters don't. This view of opposites in organizations follows the same logical pattern as that of Jung's concern for the two-sidedness of the ego, both in extrovert versus introvert personality types and in cultural expressions of archetypes. This latter idea has been developed extensively by Northrop Frye. He has identified common themes—romantic, tragic, comic, and ironic— in all literature and mythologies. Mitroff also sees organizational life in terms of these common archetypes. As Morgan says: "We are all primitives at heart, reproducing archetypal relations to make sense of the basic dilemmas of life" (1986:227). Jung's analyses are broad, including "historical, social, intellectual, and emotional dimensions...and the search for unconscious revelation" (Belkin, 1987:33).

Thus Freud and Jung tracked emotions from self to society. While Freud focused on the self, Jung went beyond and included a much broader scope. Jung developed a complex (four level) analysis of the psyche that emphasised the "cultural world of shared values." He expanded upon Freud's ideas to include the psychosocial factors. This broader perspective affected both his analysis and his interpretations. He used three questions designed to validate dream interpretations.

> 1) Are the exact details of the dream known?
> 2) Is the dream interpreted in the context of previous experiences?
> 3) Is the dream interpreted as an aspect of current experience? (Hall,1984:9).

Sociological Implications

These discussions by Freud, Jung, and others can be placed into a wider historical context to understand the emotional trauma that many patients experience. Such a perspective may include the nature of social change, from traditional society to modern society, where it is possible to separate emotions from abstract reason and where autonomous individuals exist (Homans, 1979:136). Society changed, common traditions disrupted and gave way to "a fundamental separation between public and private morality" (Homans,1979:137). According to this view, social factors produced both the theories on neurotic behavior and the researchers who wrote them.

What becomes evident is that Freud's biological determinism took a backseat to Jung's rather sociological views. The sociological aspect of Jung's work is found in his use of the "other," or complex, as it was labelled. Papadopoulos (1984) identifies Jung's concept with dialectical tradition (Plato, Hegel, Marx), but for our purposes its primary significance is found in the sociological writings of G. H. Mead. While Jung never fully developed the notion of the other, it nevertheless was "one of his central motivating forces throughout" (Papadopoulos and Saaymanurban 1984:56). And consistent with the symbolic interactionism of Mead, Jung gradually adopted the "symbol as an equivalent of the complex." Thus "one of the most significant implications of this development was the broadening of the meaning and application of the Other (as complex) by including more 'shared' or 'collective' forms of the Other....he had to move on to a new conceptual framework, i.e., the Other-as-symbol" (1984:68-69). These latter developments, however, are quite consistent with the symbolic interaction tradition, an important assumption for this study.

We learn from Freud and Jung that emotions have both biological and sociological origins. In other words, emotions are found in both our physiological nature and social experiences. These ideas have been demonstrated in the modern scientific research and the writings of brain researchers and phenomenologists. We learn from these modern studies that our emotions are more complexly arranged than previously imagined. It is by combining the insights of

Freud and Jung with the modern physical and social science writings, however, that we get the most accurate picture of human emotions. At least this appears to be the case from a sociological viewpoint.

The sociological perspective sensitizes us to the social context as an important factor in developing our treatment of clients or patients. Broad trends can influence people much more than they realize. Freud and Jung are examples of how social factors shape an individual's world view. The recent work of a British scholar named Steele provides us with an opportunity to learn just how much social factors influenced both Freud and Jung. Some of Steele's narrative analysis is summarized here in Table 2-1.

Table 2-1. Freud and Jung, Their Differences

Personal Differences	Freud	Jung
Personality	Extrovert Realistic	Introvert Idealistic
Early Experience	Conflict with Father Jew	Mystical Experience Protestant
Basic Interpretation	Biological Drives Pleasure Principle	Spiritual Destiny Religious Factors
Role Model	Scientist	Philosopher
Purpose of therapy	Find Yourself	Discover Your Destiny

Steele describes Freud as an extrovert who wholeheartedly embraced science as the only realistic and practical solution for life's problems. Jung, on the other hand, quietly clung to the idealism of the past, much as an ancient philosopher would. Jung never forgot his mystical experience as a young man, his Protestant upbringing, and the importance of religion as the source of emotions. By contrast, Freud's exposure to the Hebrew tradition both attracted and repulsed him. He was fascinated by the dreams of the Biblical character Joseph; this story obviously strongly influenced his early attempts at dream analysis. These religious roots also repulsed Freud, since the values they represented seemed to produce conflict as they were lived out through his family and with his father.

Given these differences, it is not surprising that their views about emotional health also differed. Freud believed that health is achieved as people replace both the pleasure principle and religion with the reality principle. Jung did not agree that religion was an illusion. He believed that to accept Freud's conclusion would bring disaster upon society. Without religion, the indirect, subjective wisdom of society is lost forever; replaced by narrowly direct and objective knowledge.

Their stated purposes of psychoanalysis moved in different directions as well. Steele suggests that Freud brought many of his personal family conflicts into his practice as an attempt to find himself. This would naturally guide Freud's thinking about his role as a therapist. Consequently, he saw the primary purpose of intervention to be just this: to make known to his client those forces which too often remain unknown. That stated purpose held less promise in Jung's mind than Jung's own achievement motivation perspective. Jung believed that it was those very emotions which propel us to discover our destiny. If that is the case, then a negative interpretation about emotions holds less promise for both the therapist and his client than a positive one, which would give central place to the emotional dynamics necessary for recovery from trauma.

These social differences do not minimize the importance of either scholar or his writings. But even so, what these listings help us achieve is probably worth that risk. For an analysis of this kind sensitizes us to the social-historical context from which we've come. It clearly delineates the dynamics associated with the emotional intervention that a clinician uses. Those hidden dimensions often remain just that—hidden from our view. Listen to Jung's obituary of Freud:

> Freud's psychology moves within the narrow con-
> fines of ninetieth-century scientific materialism.
> It's philosophical premises were never examined,
> thanks, obviously, to the master's insufficient philo-
> sophical equipment, but it represents a brilliant
> critique of the idealism, romanticism, sentimental-
> ity, and prudishness of the Victorian Society; Freud
> is a great destroyer who breaks the fetters of the past
> (Steele, 1982:311).

While respecting Freud's analysis and critique, Jung did not completely agree with all its implications for other aspects of social life. Based on his own philosophy, Jung objected to Freud's broad generalization; especially Freud's desire to destroy religion, art, and philosophy along with the Victorian hypocrisy about sex and human nature. Instead of doing away with religion, myths, legends, and fairytales, Jung gave central place to the basic images found within them. "Jung opposed much of the determinism of the Freudian world view, and in its place offered a nonreductive view of the person, somewhat comparable to the present-day existential position" (Belkin, 1987:32).

One's philosophical orientation does make a difference in perceptions and treatment of emotions. Perhaps that explains why Jung exploited the ideas of sixteenth century alchemists and their work on the transformation of matter. Since Jung sought any and every clue about human destiny, he found several principles in their work applicable to dream interpretation. Just as physical substances are mysteriously transformed with heat, so emotionally charged images are also transformed. In the former example, liquids evaporate; in the latter, inner images appear. These images appear in dreams, but are tied into dominant patterns of collective unconsciousness and find expression in predetermined channels that connect the inner person with others and the continuity of life.

This type of analysis obviously reflects his mystical interpretation.

To fully appreciate his reasoning, remember the kind of question that Jung asked of himself. To paraphrase, it went something like this: "Traditionally, how have people expressed those deep emotions which are inexpressible?" The answer seemed quite clear to him: by using symbols found in culture, society, and religion, images which begin to convey some of the feelings, if not the understanding, found at the deepest levels. Jung did more than present an analysis, he also suggested a constructive intervention. For these emotionally charged images have a luminous and fascinating effect upon people by impelling them to action. Since they represent ageless motives, he believed that they were not just fantasy or distortions, but images of wholeness and of significant experiences. They motivate people to discover their uniqueness and destiny, an idea not too different from self-actualization and existential philosophy. They are the creative forces which, when activated, find expression in poems, especially those with emotional significance.

Normal Behavior and Emotions

What do we learn from this type of analysis? How can it help us in emotional crises where only valid interpretations and appropriate interventions are good enough? What we see here are the social forces which shape human lives. These social differences say volumes about the two men, but they also say some things about the rest of us as well. All of us develop our personalities within the context of both past experiences and present circumstances. The intellectual foundation of psychoanalysis focused attention on both the child's imagination as it stimulates fantasies and on the adult's imagination as it cultivates destinies.

No matter where we start in our quest for human emotions—with the writings of Freud and Jung or modern writings—we end up by considering their origin. The origin of our emotions depends upon people; their release upon some external stimulation, often through another person. From birth onward, childhood impressions, adolescent disappointments, and adult resentments are indelibly linked with emotional underpinning. The exact location and intensity of emotionally laden memories vary. Some are buried deeply, inaccessible to us; others are on the surface, too close for comfort. *Emotions reflect a human quality which is sociological in nature, coming from relationships and interactions of self and society.*

Social upheavals thus provide an excellent opportunity to study exactly how people depend upon, and manage without, significant relationships. In other words, in times of crises, how do people cope? Sociologists have some understanding of how massive social changes affect daily social life. Since global and and local changes are now a fact of life, the insights gained from these studies of change are particularly important to us in our own daily lives. While the factors that propel these changes are of less immediate concern to those with losses, the effects of these changes often decrease the emotional support base for mourners. The same technology which has been used to create cities, planes, industries, satellites, and computers also increases the risk factor in life— accidents, pollution, nuclear weapons. Modern people are indeed vulnerable to hazards created in part the very instruments (science and technology) that promise to improve the quality of life (The American Dream).

No one argues that our race against time produces a "hurry sickness" which is unique to the 20th century. Its early manifestations were spotted one hundred years ago by the poet Matthew Arnold who wrote:

> Oh, born in days when wits were fresh and clear
> And life ran gaily as the sparkling Thames;
> Before this strange disease of modern life,
> With its sick hurry, its divided aims...

The clock has taken on a role in modern society even more significant than Arnold could have imagined. The classic sociological study by Alex Inkeles on modernization showed, among other trends, that modern societies do indeed compress time into smaller increments. People are hurried along in their cities, constantly racing against the clock. This is even more the case in emergency medical centers, where seconds or minutes can mean the difference between life or death. Hypertension is a disease that affects millions,including professionals in the health care fields. Eyer (1979) found that 50 per cent of those living in urban environments suffer from high blood pressure. In a cross-cultural study of epidemiology, Eyer discovered that no other explanation explains differences in blood pressure except that of social stress found in modern societies. He concludes that hypertension is endemic to our way of life; it is a social problem woven into the fabric of modern life.

Whether the crises, emergencies, or accidents are preventable or not, they do leave lasting effects on community life, for both the individual and the group. It is this interactive effect which must be taken into account in health care because it represents the nature of life in society. Using time phase in disaster research and various levels of social units, the sociologist Barton (1969) advocates multiple level classification units in diagnosis and intervention. Otherwise, the vital connection linking people together is omitted. When a flood kills hundreds of people, it also leaves behind thousands of survivors with disrupted lives. Not only did individuals suffer extreme trauma, but so did the community as a whole. With the normal social networks gone, along with their homes, the survivors experience extreme emotional agony (disorientation, apathy, hopelessness). Their social cohesiveness and neighborliness may be sustained temporarily, but resettlement destroys these even these remaining ties. So a disaster like a flood can be a double loss (physical security and moral support). The effect is to make it impossible for people to utilize their personal strength (Erikson:1976:302-305).

The Biological Basis for Emotions

The brain researcher Maclean describes three interworking "brains" in humans. Each encompasses the other, much like a baseball—core, cork, and covering. The core brain, also known as the reptilian brain, prompts instinctive behavior in people. Perceived danger automatically triggers a neural response at this deepest primitive level. In other animals it regulates behavior such as hunting and homing, fighting and mating. Maclean attributes the more complex emotional feelings of monkeys and people to the second type of brain, known as the limbic system. Experiments have shown that without this brain layer monkeys become passive and show no maternal behavior, but with it, they have the full range of emotions. The third brain is the cerebral cortex. It controls the most complex types of abilities found exclusively in human beings. These human abilities include—but are not limited to—language, culture, communication, writing, art, morality, and traditions.

Biobehavioral functions and dispositions, psychosocial affectivity and interaction, sociocultural orientation and integration—all of these are human peculiarities. "It would be a serious mistake to assume that any behavior is not, in some complex pattern of interaction, determined by all three" (Hine, 1982:). The implications seem clear: we must analyze emotions (patients or clients) from several dimensions—three, to be exact. These three are called the 3-D's: depth analysis (like psychoanalysis), dynamic analysis (like psychodynamics), and dream analysis (more like Jung in a sociological sense, but not completely ignoring Freudian input). This integrative and holistic perspective is sociological in orientation, but other dimensions are not neglected, as should be clear from this introductory chapter. This aproach is called an eclectic "3-D Emotive Theory." In a broad sense, these divisions follow the distinctions of Belkin (1987): psychodynamic, behavior, and humanistic-cognitive-group.

People express sympathy over losses, whether their own or others. What accounts for this capacity? The American sociologist

Cooley identified two ways in which sympathetic attitudes are developed: 1) through personal insights and 2) the pity or emotional feelings associated with those understandings. Discernment obviously precedes feelings of sorrow over losses (Stark, 1978).

It was another social analyst named Max Scheler who elaborated on a development sequence of thoughts and feelings with two theories. The first theory begins with the development of a person's own self understanding. As we understand ourselves and our emotions, we are better able to empathize with others in their experiences of loss. Scheler preferred a second theory that dealt with where those understandings came from. He concluded that this involved an intuitive process, not an inductive process nor even an inborn characteristic.

Scheler (Stark, 1978) did not imply that associations with others were not essential to this process of intuition; just the opposite. Without others around in close, personal, and meaningful associations, the individual has only a "well-defined consciousness of emptiness." Only in intimate relationships with others do people emotionally move toward a realization of those feelings of understanding. To love, one must be loved; and that comes as people experience love through the molding of social interaction. This second explanation builds on the reality of experienced knowledge, whereas the first one extends the idea of an analogical influence. To put it another way, the second theory goes from another to ourselves; the first theory starts with oneself and applies these insights to another.

In both theories, however, interaction with significant others is a prerequisite for the cultivation of sympathy. Both theories lead us to new conclusions about the exact linkage between one person and another. In matters of sympathy and loss, that identity of feeling springs from common experience over time. It is an intersubjective communication in which two people share knowledge, experiences, and personal feelings. Over time, these emotional memory banks are filled with both positive and negative encounters involving character traits, values, and concerns.

The Self in Crisis and Loss

It is not unusual for a middle-aged person to have experienced severe crisis in one form or another. Even those who study the phenomena of coping with the stress of loss are not immune. In his autobiography, Carl Jung openly described such an experience. When he was in his weakest mental state and emotionally drained, personal encounters with close friends and family members sustained him through the worst time of his life. Those ties of identity, purpose, and permanance stabilized his tendency toward despondency. Through these meaningful and personal encounters, people gave him the support he so badly needed.

Jung's experiences are validated by sociological studies. *These studies confirm the importance of strong personal ties during times of stress.* Hill (1965) proposed that the time for recovery after an illness or crisis is directly related to the quality of personal encounters with family members. The same principle works within any stressful environment. McCubbin thoroughly researched the relationship between strong families and recovery from a serious illness. When a family pulls together there is a significant correlation with greater chances for improvement. Personal encounters can be a most valuable resource during recovery.

Not only does McCubbin's research demonstrate the systematic effect of supportive groups, but it also points out the importance of each individual maintaining his or her own emotional well-being. There is a mutual reinforcement when the emotional stability of individual household members comes together to strengthen those less stable. Each member plays a significant role. This type of closeness is important because there are times when control is lost. According to McCubbin, the test really comes when things don't get done because of a lack of control. It is then that anger seems justifiable.

It is now believed that parents shape children's personalities more than previously believed possible. Daniel Stern, a psychiatrist at Cornell, believes that children exert their will at very early ages. When this happens at four months with eye contact, or twelve months by walking away, or at eighteen months by saying no, the positive or negative influences of the parents, he believes, are much stronger than formerly recognized.

Health care professionals who utilize emotional intervention should know the emotional state of their patients' capacity to cope. In recognizing, categorizing, and using emotional intervention, providers may use the diagram below which shows three types of losses (Figure 2-2). John Dewey originally developed these concepts to explain how an individual organizes his or her life around

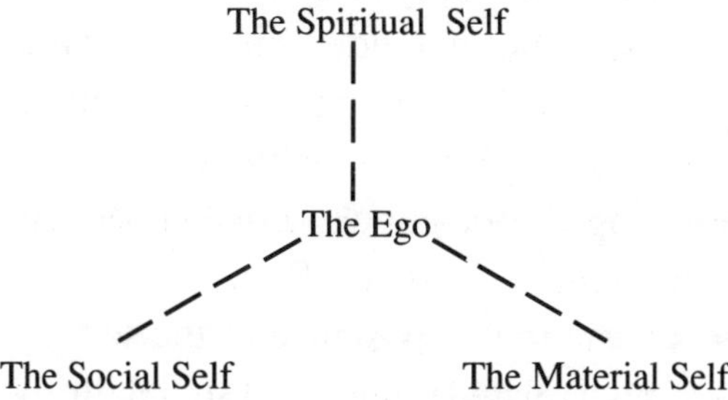

Figure 2-2. Extending Ourselves from the Ego.

various extensions of themselves. At the center is the Ego, or the active present "I am." This is where the real person resides. And it is from here that all our thoughts, feelings, and actions originate. Dewey, by comparison to Freud, did not include the id or the superego. Dewey wanted to emphasize the multiple selves which are extensions of that self.

Beginning with the material self, we should note that modern society emphasizes this aspect of the self's extension. Because rationality is given conceptual dominance, affectivity is not only repressed, but any show of emotionality is considered weakness. Thus in modern society it is not surprising to find that instrumental, functional rationality is dominant. And it is for this reason that

Freud emphasized the existence of a sphere of personal consciousness not previously recognized. According to Homans (1979:203),
Freud wanted the individual to regain control of the social order, the
second aspect of the ego. In so doing, Freud wanted to give hope to
his clients that they were in charge of their lives. Perhaps this
reflected his earlier writings in which Freud emphasized the motivation of all behavior toward goals and purposes. However, Freud
later neglected this aspect of his theory in favor of the libido
(Gaylin, 1986:48). For this reason, Homans believes that Jung
developed these ideas more than Freud. Jung not only wanted to
rescue the self from the breakdown emerging in society, but to
release the social self through means of the collective ideals and
consciousness. Jung not only dealt with the past and present
condition of the self, but extended his time frame to the future
where he hoped to provide the struggling self with realistic values.
Jung envisioned that people would achieve greater measures of self
esteem by breaking the deadlock between secular and spiritual
concerns. He thus emphasized the affective, immediate, spontaneous, sentiments basic to the existence of the self.

Doi (1986) raises a related point," that social life everywhere, not
only in Japan, is conducted according to the same kinds of rules."
His evidence comes from Mead's distinction between self and
society. Mead recognized that the way each one of us acts is from
living in relationships with others. The key ideas are: "each one
acts out" (your name), in relationship to others (job). One is
personal; the other tends to be impersonal. Doi does not mean that
this statement refutes the anthropological research on health and
illness cited in Chapter 1. His statement does not refute the cultural
themes sounded there.

The Synthesis

What we need to do is to synthesize these traditions. Otherwise
we will not balance the importance of individual factors (hardiness,
control, commitment) against the resourcefulness of social empowerment which buffers patients from anxiety. If anyone would

question the importance of the synthesis of both traditions (psychological and sociological), they should be directed to the current research findings.

Duck (1986) summarizes the health consequences of disrupted social relationships: health complaints—mental disorders, suicide—are greater for widowed men than married men. Isolated and lonely people show greater signs of depression and poor health than those with friends. Married individuals also suffer from depression if they experience separation or are dissatisfied with their partner. Disturbed relationships seem to cause the following: "low self-esteem, depression, headaches, tonsillitis, tuberculosis, coronaries, sleep disorder, alcoholism, drug dependence, cancer and admissions to mental hospitals" (Duck,1986:210).

Duck cites behavioral research which demonstrates *how social support moderates stress or illness*. Mortality is directly related to social isolation, while anxiety is inversely correlated with positive self-concepts and favorable personal relations. Those with a strong family relationship are less likely to experience psychiatric symptoms (1986:211). Some 35 million Americans suffer from high blood pressure, and emotional stability is significant for them. DeVon and Powers (1986) found that those with high blood pressure experienced not only greater health problems, but also more psychosocial problems. They demonstrated less ability to adjust to illnesses, while on the other hand, they showed greater evidence of domestic and psychoemotional disturbances.

Duck (1986) and Dawson (1986) have also found that the nonverbal cues of physicians determine whether there is open, honest communication or not. A summary of related research shows, among other things, that patients tend to interpret body signs as an important dimension of acceptance. If physicians close their arms in interviews, they are perceived as not being open or friendly; patients do not open up to them (Duck, 1986:207). Dawson (1986) found something similar. Patients first determine how the attending health care professionals will respond to them before they open up about their personal problems and feelings. If a physician leans some 20 degrees toward the patient, or if the physician smiles or nods, people think of the physician as friendly (Duck, 1986:207). Similarly, any type of physical contact can significantly affect physiological responses (pulse beat) and talkativeness (Duck, 1986:207; Dawson, 1986).

It is possible to define emotions in such a way as to underscore their relevance for health care professionals. As described above, emotion can be defined by how we feel about our past and present development. It appears that emotions are closely connected with, and emerge from, interaction with others in a cumulative fashion. Each encounter adds to the deepening layer of emotionally-ladden experiences over a lifetime.Along with each experience there is also recorded an emotional response; whenever we recall these experiences the emotions are also recalled. Those earlier images are reservoirs of feelings,along with health of body and disposition of mind. This explains the close connection between health, self, and emotions. To be healthy, then, means that the reservoir contains many emotional memories of positive greetings and encouragement from others. This pattern produces healthy emotions. The implications are obvious: well-being depends upon how we are initially and subsequently greeted, or treated by ourselves and others. Under those conditions where the greetings are full of good will, health is found; otherwise, it and physical well-being are absent.

We would expect that health care professionals can use these insights as they keep track of those charged to their care. Some of these professionals will already know the importance of this connection between emotional health and social interaction. Some patients are more neurotic in their emotional outbreaks than the average patient, but even these emotional episodes can be understood to one extent or the other. The Freudian models of emotions can help professionals in dealing with these extreme cases, while the sociological models are useful in the others. Together, these two scholarly traditions more truly represent reality than either alone. Together, they show the two-way flow of traffic between self and society, even though they started from opposite ends of the continuum. Both traditions are used to identify characteristics of emotional outbreak and development. Both traditions concern health, health care, and the patient's self image; what prevents healthy emotions and what produces healthy emotions. It is this convergence, or lack of it, that continues to capture the attention of clinicians and social scientists. Clinicians must balance the tendency to help their clients with the need to help them help themselves. Patients must learn to accept help when and where needed, but they must also learn to use their personal resources. Social scientists are concerned about what factors "lessen the chances of distress, regardless of, and without any, dependence on the level of stress. The importance of considering any and all distress-reducing factors should not obscure, however, the analytical distinctiveness of, and continued interest in, the subissue of stress-buffering" (Wheaton, 1985:354). Each of these contributions should increase the quality of health care as we rediscover both the limits of individuals and the benefits of communities. "I am convinced that we have reached the limits of individualism and our survival depends on rediscovering our need for community. In that process we have the opportunity to rediscover love" (Gaylin, 1986:243).

Chapter 3

An Integrated Theory of Emotions

Certainly one of the major concerns in the health care industry is that of maintaining quality in the face of increasing competition. This challenge may well depend upon competent professionals committed to the social dimensions of health care. Because health care is emotion laden (Chapter 1), quality care includes the stabilization and utilization of emotions in crises (Chapter 2). How then can providers synthesize these insights into an integrated theory which encompasses the full range of emotions? This chapter attempts to provide a conceptual framework for addressing these emerging concerns for quality in health care. The framework is broad enough to cover many of today's challenges in the health care field.

Since one of the crises in illness is the instability of social life (Levine and Kozloff, 1978:317-318), it is not surprising that illness is socially defined and recognized. Through acceptable social norms, the sick are excused from social participation. Even though they may not be responsible for their condition, they are nevertheless expected to return to society whenever possible. Meanwhile, professionals legitimize the person's status and chart their recovery. Some believe that the lines of demarcation for disease are still as clearly visible as they were in post war years; others suggest greater flexibility in social definitions of sickness. Still others doubt the universal aspects of such concepts as health, what is normal, and wellness.

To test these ideas, researchers should monitor the role of the sick and the relationship between physical problems and social participation. "Poor physical health may increase feelings of being rundown, feelings of demoralization about inability to function as before, feelings of hopelessness about the future, and worry about death" (Hayes and Ross,1986:397). It appears that "the link between body and mind is socially mediated, not because our bodies affect our minds by way of the social evaluations of others, but because social positions affects the shape of our bodies"(1986:398). Hayes and Ross found that physical health and activity correlated directly with income; those in low and middle income levels exercised more than those in high income levels. But to approach physical problems from a social perspective requires further elaboration. Unlike the concept of disease, illness carries more of a social recognition for both individual and group responses. It is expected, however, that as new forms of illness become accepted as legitimate, the distinction between disease and illness could well disappear.

Using content analysis to study anger and love, Cancian and Gordon found that standards of expressing emotions varied with socioeconomic periods of time. Modern norms encouraging free expression of emotions and hostility dominated popular women's magazines from 1900-1920. That trend gave way to traditional gender roles in marriage from the thirties to the fifties. Greater flexibility in gender roles dominated the seventies and eighties (1986:3). Socially accepted expressions of emotions occur in cycles, as evidenced by popular literature.

The social controls of sentiments are not only determined by broad historical trends, but also by particular reference groups to which people belong. People define illness within a social context. Customs determine what illness means and how it should be evaluated. There is a social dimension that accompanies each particular physical problem. Alcoholics and AIDS victims are evaluated differently from children with leukemia. Emotional breakdowns from stress are more difficult to explain to family and friends than physical injury from accidents.

People realize these historical and group distinctions of illness. That may explain why some illnesses go unrecognized—society is less tolerant of some physical problems than others. Based on findings at the Human Population Laboratory in Berkeley, about 35 percent of those surveyed were disabled or suffered from a serious physical problem. These conditions restricted the individual from fully participating in the life of their community. These physical problems included everything from coping with ulcers to combating cancer. Society tolerates this population group, but with definite limitations; ask any rehabilitation professional. Another 28 percent of those surveyed had symptoms that affected their capacity to assume full responsibilities. The symptoms listed were pains in the chest, anxiety over sudden changes, headaches, colds, shortness of breath, and sleeping difficulties. In spite of their physical problems, these individuals often ignored these symptoms because of jobs, family responsibilities, or other social commitments. The rest of those sampled (36 percent) were satisfied with their physical condition even though the majority of these lacked the full energy they expected (Bloomfield and Kory, 1978).

Social Definitions of Health

People who do not fit the socially acceptable definitions of illness may need to legitimate their condition. There is no clear dividing line between acceptable or unacceptable definitions of illness, between accepting or not accepting social responsibility. People in different cultures interpret emotions as differently as the language they speak.

In both the Chinese and Iranian cultures, it is felt that individuals must be protected from emotional traumas which often bring harm. These people view emotions as a "force which may be directed inward toward the self or outward toward others; which must be regulated, controlled, or contained in order not to damage the self...or disrupt social relations" (Marsella and White:1984:19). It is evident from cross-cultural studies that patterns of emotions also relate to matters of health. Concepts of emotions also influence culture and how people assess their personal health. Western concepts of emotions reflect a unique bias, attributable to Freud and his "hydraulic metaphor which views emotions as a deep, insurgent force within the individual" (1984:20). Emotions express individualism more in Western cultures than in other cultures. Emotions are one aspect of cognitive processes which operate intrapsychically.

Most Asian and Pacific cultures place emotions at the center of all social relationships. This emphasis on the interdependency of emotional linkages represents an integrated system. In contrast to the West, it is the glue of society at all levels—macro and micro, supernatural and climatic, self and society. Emotions balance all energy and cosmic forces, a view prevalent in the Yin and Yang thinking of many Asian cultures. Interpreting emotions as "sociocentric" is the basis for all relationships in most Asian and Pacific cultures. Loss of family members in some of these cultures can produce excessive emotions which also disrupt community life. Rituals allow for adequate expression of these emotions and they involve most of the community. Chinese society regulates and prevents excessive emotions; it promotes the harmony seen as necessary for good health and wisdom.

Just as these cultures influence distinctions of emotional health, so does the American culture. Since ours is a medical culture, people ask for medical opinions as much to validate their illness as to seek professional help. That may explain why 80 percent of all visits to the family doctor involve these conditions: back pain, headache, gastrointestinal distress, anxiety, and fatigue. These complaints limit social participation. They are also indexes of emotional health, since most people use physical and emotional indicators such as these to monitor degrees of emotional health.

The consideration of emotions varies with the professional specialty. Psychiatrists, clinical psychologists, and psychiatric social workers usually consider emotions to be central issues in health care, as do nurses involved with stressful illnesses or working in trauma centers. According to some estimates, the majority of those seeking emergency treatment have emotional, not physical, problems. Those most directly involved with patient care tend to be more sensitive to patients' emotional needs. If the topics listed in medical journals are indicative of interest, then the lack of articles on social and emotional factors indicates massive indifference in the medical community as a whole. Hoff believes that this neglect "does not reflect their unimportance, but rather represents a serious omission"(1984:16). The preponderance of attention to physical factors may even "obscure the highly effective group medium of helping people in crisis" (Hoff:1984:107).

After the impact of an injury, accident, or loss, health care professionals respond with surgical procedures, drugs, or other medical treatments. Yet the act itself may produce a placebo response from the patient, or a traumatic condition, making things worse. Both of these factors may influence whether a patient overcomes the crisis or not. Are these factors real, but relatively unimportant? Or do they make a difference in health care? Regardless of the answer, many of these social and emotional factors shape our lives before, during, and after an encounter with health care professionals.

The emotions of the patient drastically fluctuate during treatment. Lives are temporarily cut off from normal social encounters. If ever there were a time for personal reassurance and support, it is at this time, when the patient is under the supervision of health care specialists.

Sick people are more than biological organisms whose only need is for pharmaceutical medication; they are emotionally complex. Patients have heightened sensations, because of social expressions, extending well beyond the examination room. In an emotional crisis, the unknown and unexpected are difficult to control. Because these emotions are hard to express gracefully, they're often blurted out violently. The intensity increases with the pain of the needles, the smell of disinfectants, and the groaning of hurting people. Only the healthy professional feels at ease in this strange environment. The more severe the illness; the more intense the emotional confusion and the less of this the patient can endure. The only persons who can emotionally handle this environment are the most healthy ones—and they don't need it.

It is evident that any comparison between sick and well, illness and health should be expanded because of questions about a social perspective on wellness. Two issues—wellness as the final cure, and prevention rather than cure—form the basis for social definitions of health.

Social Life and Emotions

In 1785, Friedrich Mesmer said "there is only one illness and one cure." This is a simplistic view of health that is inappropriate today. To thoroughly evaluate the full range of human emotions is an exacting task. Sheldon Stryker (1980) has given us a valuable overview of the early writings in this field in his work on symbolic interaction. He includes the ideas of William James, John Dewey, Charles Cooley, William Thomas, George Mead, and the Scottish moral philosophers. Many of their ideas influenced the models discussed in this chapter.

By isolating the core of society, these early writers present the components of an integrated theory of emotions. A model of social life also provides information about experiences, sentiments, and emotions. After a loss, for example, nearly everyone has difficulty; we find that others become more important than before because life can no longer be taken for granted.

What theory best fits the sociology of emotions? Which concepts are the most appropriate? If we are to understand the full range of human emotions in a practical sense, let's begin with the Scottish Moral Philosophers. They proposed a similar undertaking: to develop a practical knowledge about community life. Their soundness of thought still has appeal for current social scientists who have continued that tradition in symbolic interactionism (a major theory in sociology).

From that tradition of sociology also comes an integrated theory of emotions. Those in that tradition isolated three aspects of social life: experience, sentiments, and emotions. For our purposes, these factors are essential. They are broad enough in scope to include the most relevant aspects of social cohesiveness and collective associations. These are important to include if we are to supplement prevailing thinking in health care, which has been strongly influenced by the prominence of Freudian thought about emotions. Since coping with stress is not an isolated activity, social life must also be considered. Our experience of distress is analogous to watching a sports program through the lens of either a "minicamera" on the fifty yard line or a wide angle camera on the "Goodyear Blimp." While the former gives us a close-up view of individual players, it omits other important dimensions of the game—the field of play. Just as announcers describe how the team members depend upon each other, think about how much we depend on others in patterns of life, in belief systems, and in social bonding. These three facts—habits, beliefs, empathy—are shown in Figure 3-1.

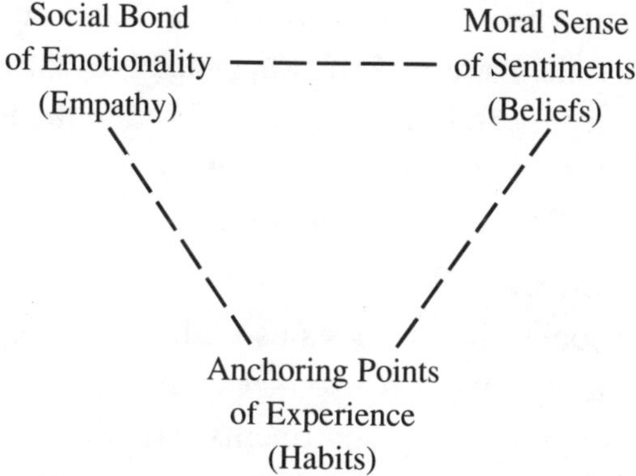

Figure 3-1. The Heart of Social Life.

Habits, beliefs, and empathy are essential for social life. Routine social patterns evolve in such a manner that we overlook their importance as anchor points of experience. Basic physical attachments—food, medicine, housing, and clothing—are the anchors. From these social anchors we obtain not only what we need but also those things we value, even our identity (Hansell,1976:31-49). These anchoring points of experience have more than symbolic significance to emotional health.

Two other dimensions of Figure 3-1 are empathy and beliefs. Our emotional state evolves from and is dependent upon our relationships with others. In the examples above, we saw that under stress a person's mental health depends upon the stability of their previous involvement with others. Everyone needs at least one person and a group with which to identify, especially in illness. Social support "moderates the long-term health consequences of the Type A behavior pattern" (Blumenthal, et al., 1987:331). It appears that social support buffers Type A persons and correlates directly with mortality (Cohen and Matthews, 1987).

Belief connects empathy and habit. People establish habits and form social bonds by the priority of their beliefs. Conversely, close personal bonds influence the moral sentiments of life. A belief about social roles influences not only the performance but also the sentiments about whether people are valued as individuals regardless of whether they are sick or unproductive. Beliefs give us meaning and purpose in life and death. Through the undercurrent values of society, these surface beliefs find practical expressions in goal setting, understanding, and motivation.

Loss and Social Life

The heart of social life provides us with the conceptual framework for evaluating loss and its corresponding emotions. Three social qualities (experience, sentiments, emotionality) form the basis for sustaining relationships. Since these qualities are the glue for social life under normal conditions, they are more significant in crisis conditions. Table 3-1 specifies what happens in losses. This table shows the impact of loss (illness, crisis, injury) on several facets of social life. The left column-experience, sentiments, emotionality-represents the undercurrents of those dynamics which shape our lives. Once these undercurrents have impacted, some changes in activities (dependent upon the severity of loss) begin to

Table 3-1. Loss and Social Life

	Disruptive Loss	
Life Processes	**Activity**	**Characteristic**
Experience	Habit	Sporadic
Sentiments	Belief	Uncertain
Emotionality	Empathy	Resentment

take place in what people do (habit), what they think (belief), and how they feel (empathy). These in turn often produce sporadic behavior, questions about beliefs, and some resentment or anger over the outcome. The more drastic the loss, the more that event disrupts the activities of life (habit, belief,and empathy).

Even rescue workers at the scene of a disaster can experience emotional problems (Hartsough and Myers, 1985:31). These workers can be stunned, as their sensibilities become overloaded. Symptoms include an inability to understand the magnitude of the disaster; some extreme cases show signs of terror, fear, horror, revulsions, and agony. In a study of over 100 disasters, these researchers found that 90 percent of all workers later recalled such feelings; 20 percent experienced severe fatigue, anxiety, and sleeplessness.

How can we apply the three elements of empathy, beliefs, and habits to the coping problems of the care givers in the health care profession? Their profession is clustered around five components of health and medical care: outreach, outpatient, inpatient, extended, and community. These can be placed into the heart of social life (Table 3-1). These five components encompass the broad spectrum of health care and are found in solo operations or health clinics (outreach), emergency treatment facilities (outpatient), hospitals (inpatient), custodial care, boarding homes, hospices, or home care (extended), and consumers, government, and professionals (community).

According to Snook and D'Orazio (1984), these five components represent all facets of health care. We could say that the anchor of experience (Figure 3-1) corresponds to the community of professionals. The other four components— extended, inpatient, outpatient, outreach—are the healthy bonds of social life. The "Moral Sense of Sentiments" is symbolized by the fact that health providers try to preserve life and render assistance in emergencies.

Professional community sentiments are the "social glue" and intensity of feelings that people have toward one another. Sentiments are what hold people together; the components include "common values," "local loyalties," "shared traditions," and "individual interactions" (Christen, 1983). Rural communities have historically fostered stronger sentiments than urban ones. Not all sentiments are lost in large cities, however, and the ones lost are offset by gains in material well-being and the quality of service expected in health care. If sentiments buffer patients in health crises and if they get lost in impersonal bureaucracies, how can a sense of community life be maintained in health care institutions? As health professionals consider quality health care strategies for emotion buffers, there's no better place to begin than with client satisfaction as an index of community sentiments.

Since the consumer's choice may determine the future direction of health care, suggestions about creating satisfaction or "sentiments" in health care service reflect more than sentimental dreams about a community life that no longer exists. When implemented, these insights about consumer satisfaction might also indicate the harsh reality of a competitive market, as the Group Health of Spokane discovered. Their membership of 26,000 increased 13 percent over the past two years because sentiments became a reality. Three goals are at the core of their delivery system: 1) socialize new members into an experience that is personal, positive, and predictable; 2) offer benefits that are clear, concise, and usable; and 3) provide total care that includes an emphasis on and support of healthy life styles. As a result, their services go beyond illnesses so that members get services whether they are ill or not.

From this viewpoint, sickness disrupts foundational patterns of social life. People normally interact on a routine basis without much thought about how important others are. Before loss, their roles (how they typically act as worker, husband, parent, neighbor) are unconsciously linked with others; what associates demand. These roles change after loss; they can no longer be taken for granted. The disruptions of loss produce emotional baggage that sociologists refer to as "role strain" or "role conflict." Because of inconsistencies in social relationships, people find themselves under some degree of emotional stress. A person becomes momentarily disoriented in times of loss. It's much like trying to bake a cake without a recipe—the guessing of ingredients itself produces some uncertainty. Even though the situation is unpredictable, the effects of this emotional disruption are predictable: layoffs, divorce, illness, and death.

The Spiral Effect

The spiral effect graphically portrays what happens to patients when roles change. The problem is one of alignment; the role ideal previously held doesn't match with the real role demands created by loss. If, before the accident or hospitalization, there were gaps between the real and ideal, those gaps become even greater. Small gaps make for easier adjustments. All of these changes produce a spiral effect and disrupt the equilibrium of patients. Each change causes subsequent changes through the three stages occurring with illness: 1) the onset of the disruption, which precipitates an identity crisis; 2) the transient stage, characterized by instability, insignificance, and uncertainty; and 3) the continuity of life stage during which people return to some stable life pattern with new roles.

There are five internal dynamics which parallel five basic questions that people usually ask. These can be seen in Table 3-2. After the initial onset of separation or disruption, people begin to question themselves. Because social relationships are taken for granted, their basic identity is in question; the inevitable question is "Who am I?" If one's identity is dependent on money, achievement, and

Table 3-2. Role Pattern Changes In Sickness

Internal Dynamics	Basic Questions
Identity	Who am I?
Instability	When is this over?
Insignificance	How can I cope?
Uncertainty	Where do I go from here?
Continuity of Life	What can I do?

influence, then there may be rather drastic changes. After the initial shock in responding to what happened, there begins a period of transience. The exact duration of this second stage varies with the seriousness of the injury or the suddenness of the event. This time can be characterized as a time of instability, insignificance, and uncertainty. It is only natural to ask questions: "When will this be over?" "How can I cope?", and "Where do I go from here?" These questions emerge from one's condition (loss and disorientation) and feelings of indifference about the instability as part of the coping strategy. If others begin to manipulate the sick person, then that in turn increases the feelings of insignificance.

In the third stage, people begin their recovery and acceptance back into society. The process of adjustment takes time, for the patient may have to struggle with role changes resulting from loss of identity due to instability, insignificance, and uncertainty. Depending upon the severity of the sickness, the patient must adjust to inconsistent role behavior: what they expect of themselves; what other expect of them; and how they ultimately act. Patients may also experience a loss of control and direction in life, at least temporarily. Instead of realizing their potential, the patients operate within a survival mode. This condition of lifelessness precipitates some thoughts and feelings about how things should or could be, but the realization seems impossible. Under normal circumstances, people worry about their status, importance, potential, supporters, and achievements. These seem less significant after illness. In their place we often find these emotions: indifference, manipulation, feelings of inadequacy, and temporalness. But what has been lost can, in most cases, be recovered; if not in fact, then at least in one's attitude.

A new life can emerge from the ashes of the old life, adjusting to reality and change. And with this new life also comes new insight about the real self discovered during times of loss and grief. After moving to this third stage of loss, patients can discover the true subject self; the self stripped of all the trappings of status, position, and power. This transformation, like the purging of a fire, leaves only that which is able to withstand the heat; it is the basic and lasting fabric of the self. If we look long enough, we can also discover love that is more basic than manipulation. Love that is unconditional and unmerited. Love that puts personal worth at the center; and underneath that is a residual of power, the power to make decisions about how we feel, how we react, and what we think. This ability to chose gives us optimism and freedom. It gives us the hope to carry on and the freedom to make our own choices. We can rediscover purpose—not as we originally planned, but as original as any planning.

This frame of reference sensitizes us to the mechanism whereby people change their status (child to adult, single to married). They do that through certain rituals such as puberty and marriage rites. *As social supports with definite cultural meaning, these activities buffer those entering into this period of changes in responsibility and status.* And there are similar changes during severe illnesses or periods of hospitalization. The social context determines not only the identity of the person but also the responsibilities. From anthropological literature, we learn about the rites of passage under normal and expected periods of transition. These insights also help us understand a similar pattern and purpose in the transitions of illnesses. Before the transition and change, a person's status depended upon both their contributions to others (achieved status) and certain socially recognized preferences (ascribed status). With disruption, the person experiences not only changes in identity to varying degrees, but also changes in expectations based on new responsibilities.

Support of Others in Crisis

We can reduce the five internal dynamics into a dialectic between identity and intimacy (Rice and Rice, 1986:83-91). This allows us to consider the relationship between support of others in crisis and the identity crisis. Intimacy involves relationships, closeness, and dependency on others; identity means separation. The former category depends upon trust, respect, empathy; the latter on autonomy and independence. This dialectic between intimacy and identity is like a rubber band; a pull on one side stretches the other; the loss of identity shifts the dynamics in the direction of intimacy.

Role patterns under the loss of identity in crisis lead to a greater need for intimacy or support from others. The person in crisis becomes confused about what is appropriate behavior. If too much is expected of a person, there is role strain. This means that there are too many activities which cannot all be accomplished. We're overloaded much like an electrical system, and like that electrical system, we too can "blow a fuse".

Another example of role inconsistency is when we have contradictory cues about what we are to do. This is called role conflict, and it means that what I think, what someone else thinks, and what I do are inconsistent. There is no alignment, but I am forced to make a decision anyway. This kind of a decision also puts stress on me. It is especially problematic when the other person is someone I work closely with or know on a personal basis.

Overcoming anxiety may depend upon well-established social systems. If these social linkages are securely entrenched, then they usually exhibit some common characteristics. Table 3-3 lists three support levels—personal, interpersonal, and intrapersonal. Good social support depends upon certain patterns of interaction. There is evidence of strong positive group support if there is positive face-to-face interaction between you and your patient; if friends come

Table 3-3. Support Levels

Analytical Category	Personal	Interpersonal	Intrapersonal
Pattern	Face to Face	Small Groups	Social Network
Prototype	I/you	Family/Friends	Physician/Counselor
Process	Assess	Validate	Examine
Purpose	Acceptance	Encouragement	Advice

for a visit; and if the network is firmly established. After an illness, the health care professional should worry about those who don't have these patterns of emotional support. Without them, the recovery can be slow and difficult.

Since caring others act to accept, encourage, and inform those of their friends in trouble, self-esteem varies directly with the strength of these relationships. When patients have few visitors, or appear isolated, it could mean that their emotional support base is inadequate. In other words, such patients lack evidence that they are "loved and cared for," that they are "valued and esteemed," and that they "belong to a network of mutual obligations" (Duck, 1986:212-213). Social facts are real in their effects, yet they are either overlooked or neglected in health care. In contrast to those without visitors, other patients demonstrate a secure, strong support system. This is achieved through significant others who give acceptance, encouragement, and advice to their friends who are patients; *they act to buffer high-level anxiety in those patients.*

Some managers and employers have formalized work place support systems in the following manner: 1) establishing groups of three to five whose responsibility is to render support whenever others experience an emotional disequilibrium; 2) using research to see what is lacking in an organizational environment; 3) encouraging all managers to develop their own skills for coaching during stressful times; 4) using team building between groups to further expand the skill base; and 5) eliminating isolation where possible by placing people together in meaningful work groups (Fritz,1984:268). This support group approach is only one way to establish an integrated view of emotions; another approach involves identifying the personal situations of people in various social roles.

Identifying Identities in Roles

To be healthy is to be growing and developing; when this stops or slows down, we start dying physically, emotionally, and socially. Physical growth is the easiest to see, but there are other aspects of growth. Growth is understanding, emotional stability, socialness—just to name a few. In the early years of our life we seek knowledge, but as adults we seek to understand. Whether young or old, the idea of roles can give us some valuable insights. We basically develop our sense of selves in the context of others. We interact with others using symbols that take on meaning in the context of a society. Values and sentiments are communicated individually from one person to another. Within these relationships we can further specify the degree to which there are primary or secondary relations. Primary relations consist of deep communications, intimate sharing, and close physical contact. Secondary relations lack those qualities.

People hold some subjective sense of who they are. That identity of who we really are influences how we behave in society. The way in which people articulate their identity becomes more problematic during times of stress. It is during these times that the real self (attitudes, feelings, sentiments) loses the anchors of social relationships. This uneasiness about who we are in turn affects how we are seen by others. Under stress, most people generate excessive amounts of emotional reactions which, if left alone, will eventually burst forth like a volcano.

It is also important to realize that our institutions tend to contain or restrict our emotional expressions. Consequently, we hold in our true feelings until we lose control or until we are in an environment where such feelings may be released. The former takes place unexpectedly and is embarrassing; the latter generally takes place at home. In the work place we can identify how the corporate culture maintains wellness and emotional health; we can then change what is not working or add what is lacking. This calls for an integrated view of emotions that solves problems, designs comprehensive programs of wellness, communicates concern, redesigns work, educates people about wellness, uses the reward system whenever possible, and counsels people for total health development along with career advancement (Fritz:1984:268).

People become confused about who they really are after the loss of a job, after retirement, or after the loss of health. Loss disrupts the stability that we once had. Until a loss, role patterns are fairly well routinized. They are part of a habit pattern: son or daughter, mom or dad, neighbor, professionals who do a certain job. All of these descriptions define roles, and in some way define us as people.

One way of explaining how role patterns work is to look at why we act a certain way. We act that way out of habit. It's the way we think of ourselves as acting. We bring to each situation certain preconceived ideas about what is or is not appropriate. Moreover, we know how other people think we should act. There are standards about the proper way to act as a parent, an employee, or a husband. Finally, we chose to act out certain behaviors that may or may not conform to what we or others think appropriate. Although each patient responds differently to disrupted health, all must struggle with shattered identities, redefined relationships, and unanswered questions. The mother's grief over a lost child differs from the father's because of how each uniquely related to that son or daughter. A mother daily meets the needs that her child has, while a father plans for the future. One is expressive; the other instrumental. One worries about baths, meals, hurts, clothes; the other deals with hikes, bikes, cars, trips. But both suffer immeasurably from anticipatory or actual grief over the loss of a child.

Recognizing the Emotional Response of Patients

For an accurate assessment of patients, you should anticipate their emotional type and response readiness. After this overview, you should have a basic understanding of patient responses. This basic knowlege needs to be supplemented with intuition, skills, and empathy. In each case you will adapt your response to the patient's. The responses of patients emerge from their outlook on life. Experiencing pain, being paralyzed, feeling hopeless—all of these emotions can block a patient's sense of direction so that the patient becomes incapable of visualizing anything beyond daily survival. Patients, like anyone else, respond to those providers who offer "emotional support, support new behavior, teach a skill, develop rapport, build self-esteem" (Howard, et al., 1987:124).

Even with a positive climate of acceptance, a patient may elect not to discuss his or her private life. That's OK—and not unusual—because they may have other outlets for their frustrations. However, as a health provider, you must be alert to patient readiness. From a development perspective, you can identify three elements of readinesss: willingness to tackle the tasks, ability to accomplish them, and confidence to complete them (Howard, et al., 1987:127). A supportive atmosphere only opens the door; the patient may still decide not to enter. The professional must be ready to assess the emotions of the patient who decides to use this door. In evaluating patients, you may want to use a compatible system like the Adaptive Counseling and Therapy (ACT) (Howard, et al., 1987). This system can be used to connect bodily responses, personality, and emotions to the social context.

The ACT model, like many others, uses the basic insights of Jung on personality types. This model reveals what constitutes the most and least effective approach to a particular patient. Some of this is based on studies of how leadership principles can be used to increase productivity. Health professionals can use some of this information effectively once they understand that the readiness level of the patient dictates the health professional's response.

There are two types of extroverted patients: "the independent doer" and "the talkative suggestor." Both doers and suggestors are highly visible, yet they differ: the doer is task-oriented; the suggestor people-oriented. Doers take initiative; they are able, willing, and confident. They resist the restrictions of medical care; if challenged, they become hostile and angry. To avoid embarrassment, realize that the doers adjust best when they are allowed more freedom than other patients.

Talkative suggestors are visibly congenial, and they take a practical approach to problems. During losses they appear able and willing, but they may lack self confidence. That lack of self confidence shows up as much in fear and restlessness as in an unrealistic and overbearing posture. These people are sensitive, gifted, artistic individuals who are good communicators. This characteristic has an advantage, for these patients can suggest practical ways to cope with their own frustrations, and are able to identify those activities that decrease fear and restlessness. More importantly, they can begin to deal with changes in their social environment as well.

In addition, there are two types of introverts: "diplomatic demanders" and "compliant listeners." They are less visible than extroverts and they differ. Like good technicians, diplomatic demanders are perfectionistic, efficient, and strong willed. They constantly hold the "stop light and red flag." Under normal conditions, they may give thousands of reasons why something won't work. Under stress, diplomatic demanders become stubborn and resistant to health care professionals, sometimes to the point of being an inflexible nit-picker. They are not afraid to speak their minds, but are unable and unwilling to show their emotions. As perfectionistic and efficient operators, they show an intolerant contempt for others. Providers should take a telling posture.

Compliant listeners, unlike demanders, will cooperate with just about anyone. This type of patient appears calm, peaceful, and cooperative. This type never complains and is always willing to comply. Yet they tend to be moody and touchy under stress. During hospitalization, they are unable or unwilling, and sometimes lacking in confidence. Their least desirable social setting is one in which nurses, orderlies, and medical staff are insensitive to their hurts and pains. They do not function well under hostile or conflict situations. When in a hostile environment, they become excessively permissive and conforming, sometimes to their detriment (Bolton and Bolton, 1984:3-28).

When interacting with patients, health care professionals should identify common patterns as clues for effectively dealing with patients. Jung noticed universal types by comparing his introversion with Freud's extroversion. It is possible to use these same insights with your patients. Some are extrovert; others task oriented. As constructed, these insights give health care workers a "game plan." Think of this analysis as a compatible system to your own. Insights from an integrated theory of emotions should also be seen as constructs applied to patients: "every person is like all other people, like no other person, and more like some than others" (Bolton and Bolton,1984:111).

Karen Horney isolated four ways to overcome anxiety: "1) affection, 2) submissiveness, 3) power, and 4) withdrawal." They can be verbally expressed as follows: "If I give in I shall not be hurt (1 and 2)," "If I have power no one can hurt me (3)," and "If I withdraw, nothing can hurt me (4)" (Bolton and Bolton,1984:153). Experienced professionals have their own way of sensing these patterns of emotionalism. And even if they operate intuitively within their own framework, the brief descriptions in the last three chapters can provide a better framework for discussing the next three chapters in Section Two: Identifying the Emotional Dynamics.

Part II

Identifying the Emotional Dynamics

Chapter 4

Sociological Descriptions of Emotions

Just 75 seconds after liftoff, the Challenger spacecraft exploded, scattering debris into the Atlantic Ocean some 18 miles from the launch pad. It was a national tragedy, indelibly etched into the social fabric of America. The sequence of events will not only be recorded with extremely accurate details, but perhaps more importantly, it will be recalled with emotional agony. Like the assassination of President Kennedy, many will recall exactly where they were when they first heard the news. Of all the responses on that particular day, the ultimate and most pressing questions came down to two: 1) Why are there tragedies like these anyway? and 2) Why do we feel the way we do? The experience and the questions really go together.

That experience forcibly broke into, thoroughly disrupted, and fully exposed the collective emotions everyone has. The reality of our vulnerability, as well as the need to collectively prevent these occurrences from recurring, was revealed. It is inevitable, then, that we ask the pressing question of "why?" Tragedies (crises, accidents, illnesses) "interrupt the flow of ordinary social life in ways that illuminate our relation to the context of our action and that show how this relation influences the experience of mutual longing and jeopardy" (Unger, 1986:174). What is most revealing, however, is that under the circumstances of social crisis, we are pushed beyond the limits of adequate expressions—even toward more practical considerations (see Table 4-1 below). It is then that we seem to need emotional expressions not normally found. With the onslaught of tragedies and disruptions, emotions become exposed, demanding immediate responses from the afflicted. That explosiveness and subsequent adjustment demonstrate how people adapt to

Table 4-1. The Social Dynamics of Disrupting Tragedy

Location	Rational/Organizations	Emotional/Communities
Externally Evident	Disruptive Roles	Remarkable Creativity
Internally Confirmed	Disjunctive Expectations	Fragmented Affectivity

their physical limitations. During a severe blizzard, the Boston City Hospital staff creatively responded in this way: 1) they teamed up to care for victims; 2) they reached out for other professionals to help; and 3) they attended to the needs—fatigue, frustration, anger, irritation, stress—of staff and volunteers (Hargreaves, et al., 1979). Other than the elderly, children, and victims, most people coped because of action to promote support, to eliminate interference, and to maintain social solidarity. All of these increased the effectiveness and efficiency of the operation (Hartsough and Myers, 1985:29,92-95).

Despite this, victims sense a double bind. Their affections are fragmented; their expectations disjunctive. Relief workers verify this. In the intrusive phase, victims may cry without reason when confronted by their fragmented and inconsistent emotions. Described as daymares or nightmares, these traumas are "difficult to identify and anticipate because they are highly idiosyncratic and may involve the entire range of sensory receptors: visual, auditory, olfactory, tactile, and taste" (Hartsough and Myers, 1985:30). Victims may deny these feelings. But denial doesn't heal. Excessive and prolonged denial (posttraumatic stress disorder) is characterized by "hyperalertness, an exaggerated startle response, sleep disturbance, memory impairment, recurrent dreams, feelings of estrangement from others, and survivor guilt" (Hartsough and Myers, 1985:30-31). Without excessive denial, Hartsough still recommends the following precautions: 1) sensitivity to the victims' emotional and mental health needs; 2) knowledge about crisis intervention; 3) the need to establish social networks in advance; 4) a definite plan of action and source of funding to provide for community needs (1982). All of this suggests the need for a sociological description of emotions.

Societal Upheavals

Neither traumatic stressors nor their emotional responses are new to city dwellers. Stress is externally evident and internally confirmed. Any urbanite paradoxically feels loneliness on freeways. Crowded loneliness runs rampant in a hurried society, and no one denies that travel affects intimacy. American Airlines serves hot meals to strangers, but flight attendants, though friendly, aren't friends. Time and technology steal intimacy not only from work, but also from home. With decreasing household size, fewer people live together. *As emotional buffers for people decrease, the whole milieu of anonymity prevails.*

Generally speaking, activities can overload our emotional capacity to endure. Social psychologists define emotional overload as the uptight, nervous, and irritable state of urbanites. Some of these daily hassles concern weight, health of family, rising prices, home maintenance, too many things to do, misplacing things, yard work, taxes, crime, and physical appearance (Brown,1986: 643-644). Several studies have shown that these daily hassles (stress) correlate significantly with somatic symptoms, disability, and visits to physicians. Specifically, stress correlates with the quality of symptoms (Norman, McFarlane, and Streiner, 1985).

Health care professionals treat not only those experiencing ill health or an injury, but also those encountering the daily hassles of life. This is true because of global and local changes and the effects of a decreasing emotional support base for those suffering loss. And this basic fact—perception of strong supporters—impacts health and efficacy of intervention (Windholz, Marmar, and Horowitz,1985).

Just as NASA engineers improve safety to avoid future tragedies like the Challenger, so too do health providers and society improve security to protect the injured who lack support. But neither group can depend upon technology alone. For the same technology used to create cities, planes, industries, satellites, and computers also increases the fear and anxiety factor in life—accidents, pollution, nuclear weapons. As one author explains, "the vastness of nuclear destruction also destroys the sense of continuity between generations on which much of the meaning of life depends"(Frank, 1984:1344; Lifton, 1979). People are indeed more vulnerable today, partly because of the very science and technology that promises to improve life.

Our focus is on how change affects emotions and health care. Implications for health care are not always clear, since describing accidents is different from specifying their impact on illness, health, and health care services. Researchers do know, however, that "a mounting literature is being accumulated on the immediate and long-term effects of disrupting human relationships" (Weiner, 1987:199-200). One example from this literature is a longitudinal study of twenty women who relinquished their babies for adoption. Researchers compared these twenty childless women with a matched control group. They found persistant psychosomatic symptoms and depression—feelings of depression, sadness, and grief—in the experimental group.

What disrupts relations may be less problematic than the effects of those disruptions on health (Condon, 1986). Studies confirm that people with distorted views of crises behave in the following manner: they give less support; they cope poorly; they solve fewer problems; and they contribute to the emotional disequilibrium (Flynn and Giffin,1984:247).

Sociologically speaking, six trends impact community well-being and mental health. These factors significantly relate to the issues of health and illness, and they can reveal some dynamics about people's response to severe losses. They address some aspects of the question about sources of illness and appropriate treatment. An understanding of these six trends, as in the Challenger incident, gives us an elevated perspective from which to visualize the social dynamics of emotions. These trends are: 1) international competition, 2) economic uncertainty, 3) cultural diversity, 4) community liabilities, 5) family instability, and 6) interpersonal inadequacies (MacManus,1986:51). Each directly impacts on health care, but for different reasons.

The first two trends (international competition and economic uncertainty) impact health care indirectly whenever workers lose their jobs and the salaries to pay for health care. These losses also mean less tax base for supporting health care research and providing public health services for the disadvantaged. The other four changes directly impact health care services, depending on the community composition.

Buffers to Societal Change

Just when small, intimate groups are needed the most, we find them less available. And just when those with losses could use some support to buffer them and mediate between them and the mass society, this support is often not there. This loss of the small group in turn affects how people cope with certain health problems which demand long-term support. These health problems, labelled "debilitating hobbles," permanently damage a person's "health." Sociologists identify them by these characteristics: strained marriage, inferior status (sex, class, race), unemployment, chronic illness, bad health, and any other impairments that permanently hinder a person's capacity to function.

With these disruptions, people experience loss of status, money, achievements, possessions, and power. Since their personal and collective identity depend upon these objects, people are unable to make adjustments without an adequate amount of grief. Letting go, giving up, and saying goodby is not easy. Such rapid changes inevitably result in an unstable environment where people may initially deny what is happening. Consequently, relations with others become quite stressful, if not already terminated. How people rebuild new relationships when old ones end may determine their ability to cope. That was the conclusion from a study where *marital support from the spouse buffered those terminated from employment* (Atkinson, et al., 1986).

From a social perspective, emotions fluctuate between the memory of what was then and what is now. Accepting new emotions is complicated by the fact that people often make the transition with fewer resources than they had before. Even their personal and collective goals must be reassessed. Coping with crises includes practical problems (bills to be paid) and social stigmas (frustrated emotions). When seeking help, people must also struggle to find just the right treatment and the best intervention strategies. Adjustment is paradoxical. On the one hand it takes time, moves slowly, and depends upon others. On the other hand, it demands quick stops and rapid u-turns. These dynamics of adjustment predispose individuals to move in certain directions, and that is where groups make a difference.

Dunn advocates the following actions to ensure that people receive quality health care: 1) improve family and community life, 2) apply health knowledge, 3) emphasize human relations, 4) develop healthy leaders, 5) influence decision makers, 6) provide creative solutions, 7) promote caring relations, 8) contribute to realistic health goals, and 9) feature those who exemplify healthy postures (Moore and Williamson, 1984:200-201). Without these counteractions, people may not adjust to changes because the "emotion buffers" don't protect them from unhealthy environments and unpleasant emotions. Job loss, for example, increases the risk for coronary failure, arthritis, alcoholism, hypertension, and gout (Cobb and Kasl, 1977; Jacobson and Lindsay, 1979; Smart, 1979). There are also serious signs of health disruption in the form of a "severely damaged environment, crumbling and loss of influence of many traditional social institutions, mortality and morbidity statistics that reflect the effects of lifestyle on health, and an alarming amount of mental illness and crime" (Stanhope and Lancaster:1984:ix).

People traumatized by divorce and injured in accidents are but one example (seen in emergency rooms) where the stresses from physical injury are compounded by emotions from social trauma. As a result, stress to emotions occurs at two levels: the social and the individual. And somewhere, between societal trends and the emergency room, is where health care professionals confront the emotional dynamics that those trends produce. How people respond emotionally is suggested by Figure 4-1 below. Ever-increasing social changes lead to fragmented relationships which in turn lead to excessive emotional baggage that can contribute to vio-

Accelerating
Social Change — — — Fragmented
                         Relationships — — — Excessive
                                        Emotional Baggage

Figure 4-1. The Emotional Impact of Accelerated Change.

lence. The rate of violence now occuring in hospitals (Engel and Marsh, 1986) has made it necessary to train staff in how to react to potentially violent situations involving patients and visitors. And this training evidently makes a difference: 3 percent of trained staff were the victims of violence, compared with 37 percent not so trained (Talbott, 1987:462).

Social Time in Loss

Loss experiences are surprisingly similar. The same intensity of time in emergency situations can also be seen in many losses in everyday life. Table 4-2 shows the connection between three factors: the dimensions of time (temporality), the events of life (pleasure) and loss (pain), and their impact on emotions. Since emotions of pleasure and pain can easily be contrasted, they are used in the table. But it is time which affects both life and loss. Each of the six responses of emotions is a function of time and event. That is, how long ago the event occurred and whether it was pleasant or painful. Depending upon the particular case, people respond emotionally, yet in opposite directions. In other words, emotions are energy levels which either lift up or pull down. It doesn't matter

Table 4-2. Emotional Responses as a Function of Time and Events

Major Events	Temporality		
	Immediate Reaction (Cueing)	**Future Responses (Releasing)**	**Long Term Impact (Linking)**
Life(Pleasant)	Heightened Awareness	Expanded Horizons	Positive Integration
Loss(Painful)	Emotional Explosion	Renewed Outburst	Negative Reinterpretation

whether the event is positive or negative, our immediate reaction (the left hand column) is to start cueing our sensors to the event. That event absorbs all of a person's emotional energy, even if they are engaged in some other activity. W can conclude that a person has emotional experiences which either expand their horizons (pleasant) or compress them (painful), as they recoil from an outburst of emotions and frustrations.

Future responses (middle column Table 4-2) pull that person inward for release either in pleasure (expanded horizons) or in pain (renewed outburst). That person involuntarily relives those events day and night, and talks again about their feelings each time they come back. Just as pleasure is integrated into life's events, so also must pain (the right hand column). The former seems easier, since the only apparent problem is preventing boredom while the person looks for another pleasant experience. With pain, however, the losers do not want to keep what they have (pain), and the winners can not keep what they lose (pain). Under normal circumstances, both emotions fluctuate with experiences and normalize with time. Once the intensity of emotions wanes, people again link their lives with others; that linkage will be a positive or negative reintegration, depending upon the type of experience (negative or positive) and the way people handle their emotions. Health care professionals contribute to this development.

Thus patients' experiences of loss force them to make major changes. Time slows as the searching continues. What seems hopeless at one time may not seem so at another. Earlier discussions about the senselessness of a tragedy may eventually give way to the need to put one's life back together. In the process, their outlook begins to change. But that change only occurs with time and the release of emotions. Looking back over the past months (or years), there is a pattern which begins to unfold. No matter who the person is, some pattern begins to unfold; cueing, releasing, and linking. With a heightened sense of awareness, the whole experience is much like a dream (or a nightmare). Those emotions grow like weeds (or flowers) and must be tended—pulled up or watered. Only then can there be the acceptance of reality and an acceptance by the patients of themselves.

Classifying Emotions

Philosophers have written about emotions since Aristotle and Plato. Despite an ever-increasing volume of literature on this subject, certain issues remain: physical connections (the speed of heart-beats when embarrassed), mental differentiation (the impact of negative thoughts and anger), particular classification (the distinction between delightful patients and others), or moral or practical implications (expressions of sympathy toward terminally ill patients). Aside from these general issues, ten questions can summarize the major analyses of emotions (Calhoun and Solomon, 1984:23-40). These questions encompass the identification and classification of emotions:

1. **What counts?** Do moods such as gloom or anxiety count along with the passions such as anger or fear? What about love? Then there is the question about whether the emotion is violent or calm. Some seem to belong to one category, such as justice, while others fit in with rage and selfishness. These aspects should be considered in formulating a definition of emotions.

2. **Which ones?** Which ones should be cataloged in certain groupings? Basic categories are most often used: positive/negative, short-term/long-term, early/late development, and forward/backward types. While most of this type of research has fewer implications for intervention strategies, there is still some merit in cataloging certain types of responses if they sensitize us to comprehensive perspectives on emotions. This is not to say, however, that it is necessary to describe a full range of responses, since so many basic categories have already been created by past researchers.

3. **What for?** This question suggests some issue about intentionality or purpose. Since emotions have objects toward which they are directed, it seems logical to include some discussion about those objects; whether they are people, situations, God, or material objects.

4. **How useful?** That is, what do emotions explain? Are they connected to physiology or the mind, or both. If we say that someone is angry, how useful is that explanation? If they get angry enough to exert influence in a social sense, then there is some logic to such a state of mind.

5. **Why rationalize?** If emotions are nonrational or irrational, then how can we begin to rationalize them? They may be neither, but their effect can be plainly observed.

6. **What's right?** Beginning with Aristotle, ethics and emotions have been tied closely together. Some philosophers connect emotions of sympathy and sentiment to ethics and morality. In the Christian tradition, some emotions such as faith, hope, and love are elevated above others such as pride, anger, and envy.

7. **Whose culture?** This issue revolves around the corollary question of instinct and environment. Are there universal emotions which transcend all cultures? Or are emotions determined by culture?

8. **How expressed?** How do people usually express their feelings? Some people use nonverbal means, while others verbally

show their emotions. What is the connection between cause and effect here?

9. **Who is responsible?** The issue here is akin to the legal debate over insanity. Are people victims of their rage and therefore unable to control themselves—"that's just the way I am." If emotions are seen as instincts or physiologically determined, then how can people be held accountable for their own actions? On the other hand, if emotions are tied to beliefs, then there is some measure of individual and group responsibility.

10. **Where is knowledge?** Does our knowledge about these various issues regarding emotions give us the capacity to change them? If what a person believed would happen under medical supervision did in fact determine how they responded, then—if they later find out that information is incorrect—how does such knowledge affect them?

Asking these questions suggests that oversimplified descriptions will not do; emotions are as complex as the person who expresses them. The fact that patients prefer anecdotal or journalistic stories to scientific descriptions of emotions shouldn't surprise us. Sociologists use dry scientific language to explain how emotions affect patients, but writers use prose that is charged with the electricity of human emotions. Marcel Proust in his *Cities of the Plain*: "The time which we have at our every disposal is elastic; the passions that we feel expand it; those that we inspire contract it; and habits fill up what remains."

Many classical writers of the last century—William James, Max Weber, and Emil Durkheim—wrote about emotions. They left several questions unexamined, however. They did not tell us how much our passions distract us, or how little our minds guide us. Those questions were raised by contemporary scholars and have direct implications for well-defined categories and multi-purposed methods used for analyzing and understanding emotional responses to life situations.

It is not the purpose of this chapter to evaluate the classical, nor even the contemporary theories on human emotions. And yet the insights resulting from some of those theories could help some individuals understand and cope with their emotions. Those same individuals could then select a patient-care method different from the ones now used. There are times when patients become discouraged; we forget that care is also necessary to cure. Emotionally caring is equal to curing; if not in the market place, then at least in the realm of motivation. By extracting those issues, definitions, and parameters of emotionality, perhaps people can utilize these ideas in order to construct an appropriate model of care.

Preferred Methodology

Those professionals who observe the devastating effects of emotions may begin to regard the feelings of their patients to be as important as the medicine that is prescribed. No one denies that emotions are real in their consequences; women, for example, who experience a stillbirth need extra care and support. Rarely do providers confront such situations without realizing the importance of support. To understand emotions is to be able to provide patients with valuable information. Providers, along with behavioral scientists, ask probing questions about the source of emotions. Do they emerge from specific situations or from innate human qualities? While arguments exist for both perspectives, it seems that particular situations and innate dispositions shape emotions into a complex mixture of both. In developing a theory of adjustment to illness, providers could use insights about how people are socialized to express their emotions. Consistent with a particular society, people develop qualitative distinctions between certain sentiments. These sentiments then provide the framework from which people learn to see their world. And that process of learning is called socialization. A child is socialized to internalize these qualitative distinctions between certain sentiments. Once socialized, these unconscious, yet distinct, sentiments determine how people interact and how they view such interaction. But more important for health care is how expressions and feelings are controlled by certain groups or individuals. This distinct classification of sentiments predisposes patients to express them not only in socially acceptable ways, but also through conventional means (Scheff, 1983).

This particular view, situationally specific level of analysis, is useful for health professionals. It does, for example, help us understand the former practice of isolating terminally ill patients from their families. This was accepted procedure just a few years ago. Now, however, not only are hospitalized patients allowed to see their friends, but some patients even come and go from the hospital for their treatments. There is much greater flexibility in providing health care now than just a few years ago. The process of changing both the perspective and the procedures took time, suggesting that conventional norms are real but invisible standards of behavior.

Universalists, in contrast with situationalists, view emotions from a biological perspective. They believe that emotions emerge from genetic factors which prompt similar expressions regardless of the setting. Several researchers have analyzed different cultures, primitive and advanced, to determine whether such basic emotions exist. They found that variation of culture does not affect some emotions—happiness, anger, disgust, sadness, and fear/surprise (Scheff, 1983:342). These studies appear to support a universal view of emotions.

Some authorities suggest that both situations and dispositions shape emotions. Beyond shaping, there is another question: what aspects of the individual are affected? Do emotions occur in the mind or in the body? Universalists argue for body-centered emotions. They locate the universal character of emotions somewhere other than in the mind. To them, emotions are in the body because they are not determined by social situations. Similarly, situationalists argue for mind-centered emotions. If society determines how people learn, then people learn standards of behavior before they express their emotions.

Not surprisingly, the medical profession tends to locate emotions within the body; recent developments, however, have tilted that trend in the opposite direction—toward mind-centered emotions. It may be useful to see how social developments in medical care affect the explanations of emotions—whether viewed as obstacles to healthy recovery or as stimuli for new life styles. But to argue for one or the other may not be the most profitable course for health care professionals; there is another type of resolution which holds greater promise for those charged with health care—an integrated approach. One prescription along this line is the scholarly approach of Scheff, a work of synthesis and exposition,not of analysis or discovery (Scheff, 1983).

There is evidence to suggest that an integrated approach may be the best in identifying the emotional dynamics of people. Scheff (1983:347) cites a study in which Japanese and Americans watched films designed to elicit emotional responses. By monitoring their emotional responses (using a hidden camera), researchers observed how Japanese reacted when alone and in the presence of other Japanese. The expressions of emotions varied less for Americans than for Japanese, who have strong group norms. These findings support an integrated approach to the study of emotions. When viewing the film alone, Japanese showed emotions similar to Americans, but Japanese in the company of others responded differently from Americans—smiles replaced their frowns. These adaptations of emotions are best explained if theorists integrate both explanations: situational/universal and mind/body.

Measuring Emotions

Researchers need an intellectual climate that challenges their thinking. The order of ideas discussed earlier does that. From the variety of questions asked above (1-10), it is evident that emotions occupy a significant place in the issues of life. Earlier scientists (medical fields) limited their attention rather narrowly to either physical responses or social settings. Consequently, the topic of emotionality was given secondary, not primary, treatment. That trend toward rationality has only recently changed, with the addition of significant criticisms and extensions to this earlier emphasis. Denzin (1984) clarified three useful assumptions for studying emotionality: 1) emotions should not be considered incidental to life itself; 2) emotions should not be studied as if they were static entities; and 3) emotions should not be evaluated by the natural science method of causation.

Beyond these assumptions, Denzin recommends a strategy for observing emotions. He advocates the use of dynamic concepts which sensitize us to "emotion-as-a-process." Because emotions possess an expanding nature, analysis requires introspective understanding. We must never mistake the methods that are funnels of knowledge for the phenomena that are well-springs of life. As for methods, Denzin includes case studies, historical accounts, myths, and fiction. All locate emotions in personal biographies where people adjust to the losses of life.

Because so little is known about emotions, Denzin (1984) himself shifts back and forth from records of personal accounts to writings of contemporary authors. This interactive approach increases the accuracy by which people describe and understand how emotions work. Most of his ideas come from behavioral sources which combine insights from a variety of other areas: case studies, literature, and religious experiences. By mixing these sources, we should be able to gain greater insight about loss experiences.

Research literature records at least three classification systems: developmental, behavioral, and physiological. The third classification is covered later; the other two, developmental and behavioral, are presented here. Developmentally, emotions begin with newborns as they differentiate nonverbal sending emotions (Buck, 1984). Within the first 36 hours, newborns will respond to the facial expressions of adults. Adults who make happy, sad, or surprised faces find that babies mimic them. Within six months, babies show signs of distress, delight, anger, disgust, and fear. At 12 months, they express their own emotions toward adults. By two years, new emotions—jealousy, joy, frustration, anger—appear both in variety and frequency of display. These emotions spontaneously express themselves on the face or in the body. They also mirror the social and cultural context. Two-year olds, getting their first vaccines, feel pain and show it by crying. That crying is spontaneous and without reservation. Only later do children learn to control pain. Control of emotions and trust in others not only prepare children for organizations, but also demonstrate that innate ability precedes social learning. Studying developmental cycles of emotions thus begins with naturalistic observations, continues through nonverbal communications, and culminates in social interactions.

It is difficult to find emotions in the mass of social science materials; some are tempted to avoid them. Behaviorally speaking, there is a way to find these emotions by using the work of the French psychoanalyst Jacques Lancan.   He follows the clinical tradition in writing about the individual's earlier experiences, which are deposited in the body (Denzin, 1984). Not unlike G. H. Mead, Jacques Lacan describes the subjective self as a perception of others' perceptions. People come to see themselves in very much the same way that they are seen. By exploring personal memories, social rituals, and family traditions, Jacques Lancan isolates and identifies the influence of others. He also explores the total stream of experiences that ultimately determines the capacities and limitations of emotions.

Of more practical concern is the research by Hochschild (1983) that exaimined the work experiences of stewardesses. She suggests that women must learn to pretend or play by the rules at work. They are not able to express their true feelings. In our society, spontaneous expressions are culturally and economically dominated and controlled. People separate their true feelings from those they present to others. About a third of American jobs require substantial emotional labor of this kind. The employee must learn to hide true feelings in order to please the boss; to reveal them is to risk rebuke.

Both Lacan and Hochschild demonstrate such complex issues of emotions.

Reviewing the behavioral literature, Denzin (1984) identifies one of the more innovative writers on emotions. Collins developed the marketplace theory of emotions. In that theory, he describes emotion as an exchange paradigm. The interaction of people is embedded in the sentiments and traditions of society, meaning that emotions are ritually controlled and exchanged by customs and traditions. The marketplace of society, then, determines how emotions are expressed. Such a view places emotions in the mainstream exchanges of life, where they are regulated. Lacan and Hochschild would agree with Collins that emotions, like sentiments, are a social phenomenon.

Connecting Patient Care with Emotional Dynamics

The medical perspective is the final example of a classification system. Various selections here are from Dr. Lynch's work and the Psychophysiological Center at the University of Maryland Medical and Nursing Schools. That team of medical specialists is interested in how patient care affects emotions. They observed how patients responded to verbal encouragement. Based on the work of Lynch, it appears that those individuals who live alone have a higher probability of premature death than those who live with others. After validating these findings, Lynch then tried to explain them. He asked two questions: how exactly does isolation affect those divorced, widowed, or never married; why does this social factor seem to produce higher levels of premature death? To pursue these questions, Lynch measured the physiological responses of hypertensive patients as they interacted with their therapist. His measurements and the theories of Pavlov gave him some answers. Isolation affects the heart because despair leading to premature death is a medical reality, not a poetic myth (Lynch, 1985:69).

Using sophisticated laboratory equipment, Lynch attempted to measure the mind and body responses. Specifically, he wanted to know how struggling heart patients survived. What physiological affect do these factors have on heart beat and rhythm : 1) visits from wives or friends, 2) touch of a nurse taking a pulse, and 3) interaction with the therapist. Since 1969, his team has recorded how significant the presence of others can be for body responses. Lynch believes "that both hypertensive and migraine headaches can be thought of as a form of internal blushing; and that since others cannot see these vascular changes, they cannot help a person identify the emotional meaning of his or her bodily reactions" (Lynch,1985:224).

Evidently, language affects the heart so drastically that it can be considered lethal. A striking, even terrifying, illustration is recorded by Dr. Brown, Professor of Cardiology, Harvard University School of Public Health. The incident involved a hypertensive heart patient who mistook the words "this woman has TS" to mean terminal situation, not tricuspid stenosis as intended. After making this pronouncement, Dr. Levine abruptly left the hospital. It was up to Dr. Brown, then a postdoctorate fellow, to correct the patient's misconception. The patient remained unconvinced up until the time of her death from massive pulmonary edema. The physician's words, even though misunderstood, literally frightened the patient to death. "To this day, the recollection of this tragic happening causes me to tremble at the awesome power of the physician's word" (Brown, 1984:14). In contrast to that woman, Dr. Brown observed another patient who, though critically ill, recovered remarkably. That patient gave this account of his experience to his physician: "You listened to my heart; you seemed pleased by the findings and announced to all those standing about my bed that I had a wholesome gallop....I figured I still had a lot of kick to my heart and could not be dying. My spirits were, for the first time, lifted, and I knew I would live and recover" (Brown, 1984:15).

Lynch's research led him to believe that what the care giver says was vitally important to how the patient responds. That relationship resides not merely in the mind or the body, but somewhere between patient and the professional. "Human feelings occur between human beings as well as within individual bodies" (Lynch 1985:271).

In a study of 27,779 adults with cancer, other researchers substantiated the work of Lynch. Some (23 percent) were less likely to die because of social support, higher joint income, earlier and better treatment. This medical team found many indications of social support linked to lower risk; the married are 19 percent more likely to detect cancer before it spreads (Goodwin, 1987).

Noncompliance may also depend upon the quality of the relationship between the physician and patient. Emotions flow easier if there is trust. In a trusting relationship, patients will more likely express their needs, wishes, and emotions. Berg (1987) concludes that empathy (quality relations) correlates directly with compliance (accepting professional advice).

In a study of a rural community of 399 Canadians, there was an even division on what was expected of a medical doctor. Fifty percent of those surveyed worried (anxiety, depression, sleeplessness) about life changes and wanted more than physical involvement. They looked to the doctor for understanding, referrals, and treatment of their emotions. The chronically ill also appear to need and benefit from quality interaction with others. A study of 450 patients with hypertension found that some controlled both their emotions and blood pressure. They controlled hypertension not with medication, but by these techniques: problem solving, having friends, and eating the right food.

People not only actively distinguish their body feelings, but they also consciously adjust to those feelings. Yet Freud did not logically cope with his own cardiovascular distress. There is an "interplay between emotional experiences, the nature of human feelings, and dynamic shifts in his own cardiovascular system" (Lynch, 1985:294). Since Freud did not fully understand the interactive effect of these factors, he was unable to accurately detect the full impact of his own feelings on his health. "It appears likely that he had the very same alexithymic problems (the inability to feel his own feelings) that plagued virtually every patient described in this book....Freud had a hyperreactive cardiovascular system that he could not feel, and thus he would have been unable to gain insight about episodes or interactions that triggered major stress reactions inside his body" (Lynch, 1985:295).

Lynch reached three conclusions about his research on emotions: 1) human interaction and health are an important part of the daily events of life and it is in this broad context that health really begins; 2) since there is an interaction affect between mind and body, reason and feelings, we must seek to understand both; and 3) the medical team should not only acknowledge human crying and suffering, but also regard these emotions as friends. After all, medical staff have the same feelings and should recognize, in themselves as well as in others, the importance of these emotions. Only through these means will any of us respond to the needs of others and share with them as human beings (Lynch 1985:310).

And only human beings have that capacity; technology doesn't. Medical technology is used to eliminate some of the emotional trauma of diseases, life chances, and surgical procedures. But despite these improvement, its influence is secondary to such factors as social conditions, public health measures, and personal behavior. The emotional dynamics of health and care suggests that attention be given "to the more complete social and psychological being," not to exclude "social roles," "mental activity," "emotional state," "a sense of well being and relationships with others" (Levine, 1987:4). *An emphasis on quality health care should result in improved health practices which, in turn, serve to buffer the emotions of patients.* This outcome is true only as professionals evaluate "health intervention in general, and medical intervention in particular" (Levine, 1987:3) in light of this standard of quality.

Chapter 5

Destructive and Constructive Outlets to Emotions

On December 5, 1987, family members stood outside the federal prison in Atlanta. Although these people gathered as one, they actually belonged to two groups: families of either the 89 hostages or the 1,105 inmates. Ironically, it wasn't force that quelled the riot and lead to a settlement. The solution to the hostage take-over and stalemate came from an unexpected source. No one expected a quiet soft-spoken man like Augustin Roman to calm those frustrated inmates. Bishop Roman could empathize with their feelings; emotionally, they were compatible, and that was the basis of communication—feelings. He allayed inmate fears not only this time in Georgia, but at an earlier time in Oakdale, California. Expressions of emotions are not always predictable; yet this time constructive emotion prevailed.

In contrast to hostage takeovers, the routine and uneventful patterns of social life hide the full range or meaning of emotions,constructive or destructive. People learn to control their emotions, and even caregivers may feel uneasy about any expression of true feelings. It is only as patients talk about their feelings that they work through grief or loss. This is why hospitals organize support groups to assist patients emotionally: prenatal loss groups, ethics committees, AIDS task forces, terminally ill patients, and critical care units. It is possible, however, for caregivers with low tolerance for anxiety to misunderstand the meaning of expressed feelings. Dugan (1987:25) cites one study where students observed, then interpreted, such expressions from a leukemia patient. Those observers with high anxiety levels evaluated the responses (video interview of the patient) differently from those observers with low anxiety levels. The first group projected their own anxiety onto that of the patient and described her as anxious and depressed, an inaccurate assessment. If caregivers can mistake emotional states, then what about patients?

Patients feel the impact of emotions in emergencies: heart attack, automobile accident, serious burns, breathing problems. At such times life is suspended by a single thread. Nobody knows the boundaries of life better than resuscitated patients with near-death experiences. Sometimes these "near misses" are later retold; other times they aren't. It's only later, after the experience, that patients explain how the emergency happened and what it meant to them.

Which is worse, a sudden emergency caused by an accident, or a gradual one brought on as a disease overpowers the body's ability to resist? That is an important distinction, since both kinds of disease are found in health care. The example of a gradual disease has taken on new emphasis in the current AIDS crisis. According to the Surgeon General, AIDS is both a life-threatening and public health problem which produces lingering emotions of grief, especially traumatic with its attached social stigma. According to estimates, 270,000 people will be affected by 1991, and of that number, 145,000 will need health care estimated to cost from 8 to 16 billion dollars (Koop, 1986:2783). While the subject of emotions was not considered in this report, the cycle of pain, anxiety, insomnia, stress, and depression is all too evident.

Endometriosis is a disease that may not be as deadly as AIDS, but it is a major cause of infertility which affects nine million women. This gynecologic disorder involves a number of painful emotions: dilemmas of surgery, effects of medications, and pains of severe menstrual cramping. Women with these emotion-laden experiences often withdraw from others (Stein,1987:168). Some, however, learn to live with pain, infertility, and sexual difficulties. For many, the emotional stresses caused by a diagnosis of endometriosis lead them to seek professional help.

All of us seek the help of a health professional some time in our lives. The request may not always be as dramatic as the cases just discussed, but they are all legitimate requests dealing with potential health problems. Each problem carries its own emotional baggage, some constructive and some destructive, depending upon the person. Since much of the interaction between provider and recipient carries emotional overtones, this chapter describes the emotions connected with health care. These heightened emotions give that event personal meaning, and even its value and interest. These life experiences either motivate people in the search for recovery or depress them in their illnesses.

The Sick Role Dynamics

If emotions have constructive and destructive outlets, then quality care means transforming the destructive outlets. Professionals do that when they plug into their patients, like conduits, and allow them to express themselves freely and openly. Through another person, patients find not only release from their losses, but also purpose for their existence. Both occur in a social context. Sick patients need emotional support for releasing their tensions, fears, and anxieties. And the human conduit comes from one with similar emotions such as compassion, sensitivity, and acceptance. As for one's purpose for living, that too involves a significant other, one who is trustworthy. Whether for release or reassurance, people define the sick role and its social dynamics.

These dynamics of sickness occur in a social context. Researchers have for over 25 years taken that social context seriously. They have identified the process of change which occurs in sickness, and it is this information which also identifies the flow of destructive and constructive emotions. Levine and Kozloff (1979) have synthesized that information, beginning with "normal," into five stages:

1) Wellness is defined from both the physiological and sociological viewpoint to include a socially comprehensive definition. This is the stage before the injury, sickness, or

surgery. As such, it forms the baseline from which everything else is measured.

2) Next comes the transition stage into the "state of illness, disability, or impairment" (1979:319). It is here that changes occur which begin the process of redefining.

3) Then comes the coping stage, with the negative impact of pain, irritability, and performance problems. If stage two begins the full range of emotions, here is where it gushes forth. Health care workers can provide a great deal of emotional support during this period of stress.

4) After some time spent coping with stress, the patient learns to play the new social role. This change appears as the patient adjusts to new expectations, both individual and collective. With these adjustments, the patient learns how to manage emotional release by asking numerous questions: What's acceptable? What's not? Who cares? How can I continue emotionally? "Depending on a number of factors (severity, chronicity, cultural values, self-conception, relations with significant others), the new role may be a predominant part of the person's behavioral repertoire, or role set; or it may be quite circumscribed as to the settings and length of time in which it is played" (Levine and Kozloff,1979:320).

5) These stages finally lead to either recovery from the incident and its effects, or continued dependence upon others. The role dynamics also change with this last stage. When there are chronic problems or terminal illnesses, that in turn determines how many destructive and constructive outlets are needed. In severe disruptive cases, the intensity of emotions probably runs higher than in less severe cases.

These stages, however, also depend upon both the event and the person so affected. The emotional transition from normality to sickness varies with the nature and severity of the impairment:

physical disability, chronic and terminal conditions, alcoholism, pregnancies, mental illness; and other factors such as social class, occupation, sex, age, ethnology, and religion (Levine and Kozloff, 1979). Emotions also vary with certain moderating characteristics of those affected. Destructive emotions have less effect on those individuals with high measures of the following characteristics: self-esteem, time management skills, change skills, assimilation of information, assertiveness, positive feedback, physical activities, finances, and peer facilitation (Clark, 1986:326-332). These are important distinctions, because they further identify the causes and effects of emotional instability, often referred to as the loss syndrome.

The Loss Syndrome

Any emergency paramedic knows that dreadful happenings can come from anywhere without warning. But even with a warning, people are never quite ready for the devastation that follows. The emotional cycle that follows is the same in kind if not intensity for all emotional losses. Whether it was expected or not, people show stress from severe crises: heart attacks, automobile accidents, stolen property, loss of friends, violent attacks, severe storms, natural disasters. Were these events and their subsequent impact all that the victim and the health care provider had to cope with it would be difficult enough indeed, but there is more to these crises than that.

After a crisis, the patient replays not only the event, but also the emotions felt during that event. General anxiety, sweating, dizziness, and palpitations can be part of this. Some people even "feel strange" because they have an apprehensive expectation of the worst. They exhibit excessive worry, edginess, and impatience. They are irritable long after the event itself. To replay the traumatic events is to relive the emotions associated with those events.

What are we to make of these disturbances? How are they recognized? What do they mean? The loss syndrome drescribes the effects of loss and grief and provides a frame of reference for patients as they adjust to change. We measures how patients respond, the various stages of that response, and learn how to recognize those stages. Once manifested in the first encounter, the impact has a ripple effect through all the other stages.

Words alone fail to fully capture the emotions. Words describe emotions, but no words can adequately convey what is happening inside the person. It would be impossible for another person to experience the same intensity of feelings even if they had had a similar crisis. Table 5-1 shows the association between phases of loss and their concomitant emotions. While representing the full array of possible responses, these emotions may not occur in just this way or even at all in every instance. They have been reported, however,in a variety of studies.

Table 5-1. Severe Loss and Associated Emotions

Phase	**Emotion**
Shock	Numbness, Disbelief
Disorganization	Despair, Fear, Franticness
Searching	Yearning, Weeping, Restlessness
Grief	Fatigue, Depression
Letting Go	Guilt, Shame
Separation	Anger, Anxiety
Resolution	Relief, Peace
Reintegration	Acceptance of Loss, Action

The loss of a parent is an example of a loss common to persons in all cultures. As we begin to accept life without the parent, we gradually move through the various stages until we experience what some have called "a ray of hope in the midst of darkness." But that progression is not easy. After a few days of shock we still can not believe what has happened. Next comes uncertainty, as we search for the recovery of what was lost. We grieve throughout the ordeal, and only later do we begin to let go, separate ourselves, and say goodbye to the lost parent. Emotional equilibrium is reestablished, but only after much struggle. It is the secure ones with self-esteem, change skills, positive feedback, physical activities, and peer facilitation that adjust best.

What about those with low self esteem who are already overloaded emotionally? People with serious personal problems who lack social support are at high risk for suicide or for rapid physical deterioration. Other symptoms associated with severe loss include: exhaustion, burnout, stress, illness, denial, and passivity. With the present day decline in family and community support, some may not know when others are hurting. Many households have become isolated from community support. As a result, they lack the emotional support to adjust or to change; they experience more difficulty with the loss syndrome. The notable exception to this is a national disaster such as the Challenger tragedy, which draws the community closer together.

Losses neutralize gains that people have made. Those achievements seem less important after the loss. People broaden their horizons when their emotions oscillate immediately after loss; their sense of ultimate worth changes. Out of control emotions and unpredictable moods change like the weather. And just when people think they can predict their feelings, they're as wrong about their predictions as the weatherman often is. Rarely has a scholar isolated the issues of loss as succinctly as the cultural anthropologist Ernest Becker (1975:IX). Just before his death, he wrote that the idea of death haunts us so much precisely because in it we are confronted with the final loss. Consequently, people stay busy. That business "...is a mainspring of human activity designed largely to avoid the fatality of death, to overcome it by denying in some way that it is the final destiny for man."

Losses in life have a way of jolting people back into the realities of social life. With each loss in life, people are reminded of their frailties and inability to cope. Becker expressed the dilemma this way: "The irony of man's condition is that our deepest need is to be free of anxieties of death and annihilation, but it is life itself which awakes it, and so we shrink from being fully alive." That shrinking is more profound immediately after a loss. The loss syndrome is a physical manifestation dependent upon social life. To know others with similar experiences helps. Left alone, people with loss experience more bewilderment and confusion. Issues and perspectives get blurrier. Friends listen, but counselors give direction. Yet all feel lost at times; therefore, they need guidance through these difficult times.

Exploding Emotions

If not controlled by society, emotions create added misery for people. For once unleashed, these inner passions overwhelm social order; this in turn can lead to violence. It is frequently asked why seemingly ordinary people show such destructive and constructive emotions. Yet 86 million people suffer from chronic physical pain which also produces erratic emotions (Feuerstein, et al, 1987:425). To ignore exploding emotions is to overlook the growing volumes of relevant research on human emotions. Emotions are not just abstract concepts which philosophers use to debate questions about human nature. Emotions are also unpredictable empirical realities which move in opposite directions, constructive and destructive. Destructive emotions can have many outcomes: battered wives, abused children, non-accidental injuries, murderous obsessions, traumatic depression, and violent families (Kemmer,1984).

Constructive emotions are found in strong families. These families have positive characteristics: commitment, appreciation, communication, time, spiritual wellness, and coping ability. Stinnett and DeFrain (1985:14) identified these six qualities in strong families: 1) They promote and emotionally support each other; 2) They affirm one another; 3) They frequently communicate on a regular and positive basis; 4) They value quality time together; 5) They possess a higher commitment; and 6) They emotionally support one another in crises and stress.

Strong families represent only one example of constructive emotions, and emotional crisis represents only one example of destructive emotions. Lifton studied and identified the emotions that follow severe trauma (prisoners of war, atomic bomb survivors, major natural disasters). In such events, people exhibit these emotional stages: 1) numbing, 2) imprinting, and 3) bearing. By "numbing" Lifton meant that people initially lose all sense of emotions. It is as if their nervous system were severed. Then the "imprinting" stage follows, an experience whereby people recall over and over again what happened to them. These recollections are cognitively traumatic, and they also produce the emotional symptoms which make it more difficult for a recovery and return to normal life. It is in the "bearing" stage that people have problems with survival guilt. They begin to ask questions: "Why was I the one to live?" "Why me?" And these questions produce guilt feelings. Lifton's research has resulted in several suggestions for learning how to deal with these emotional stages:

1) With numbing, know what to expect and visualize yourself in an objective, detached manner.
2) With imprinting, expect difficulty in adjustment. This can help to limit the build-up of additional emotional strain.
3) With guilt, anticipate and decide to cope with meaning and purpose in life. It will eventually happen, so begin to think about it beforehand.

These suggestions and insights should help not only the victims, but the caregivers as well. From Jung's views on types comes an emotional profile of the reactions of patients. Figure 5-1 is an attempt to diagram the dynamics of excessive emotions. Patients cite an event which leads to an implosion within them. From that point on, their emotions fluctuate back and forth from love to hate.

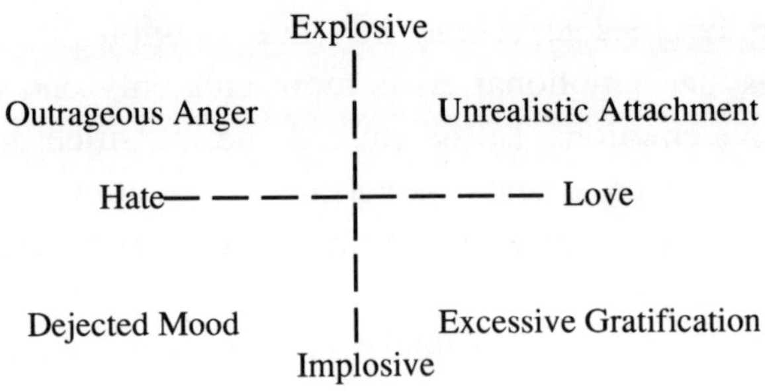

Figure 5-1. Dynamics of Excessive Emotions.

This model uses some of the ideas of Hine (1983), who formulated an integrated theory on the psychodynamics of neurosis. In his model, as in Figure 5-1, the center reflects a healthy, flexible person who is motivated by a balance of behaviors. Once that healthy limit is exceeded, then interpersonal problems begin. Our model diagrams emotions of interpersonal relationships much like the clinical work of Hine (1984) and Denzin (1984), who connect emotions with violent and nonviolent (modulated) behavior. Violence is the discharge of emotions. It is directed toward someone or something that has produced the distress. An imbalance occurs for any number of reasons, but the result is the same: a dejected mood slanted toward the object of hate. Not only is hate balanced between the emotional dynamics of outrageous acts (anger) or rejected feelings (mood), so is love. Love can fluctuate between excessive gratification and unrealistic attachment.

Our model (Figure 5-1) uses implosive-explosive emotions for Hine's dominance and submission. Both models imply that there are normal, healthy ways of coping, as well as abnormal, unhealthy ways of coping. As a professor of psychiatry (Duke Medical School), Hine has done extensive work in classical psychodynamics, consolidating the contributions of nearly 100 years of research in that field. Our model shows how people handle their emotions in stressful circumstances of loss or illness. The vertical axis and the horizontal axis both show important aspects of the individual's reaction to crisis: direction and intensity of feelings.

A little girl returned from the county fair and described her experience on a carnival ride: "Dad, do you remember that last year I was afraid of riding 'the octopus'. Well, this time I rode it with Betty. After we paid for our ticket and waited our turn, we were strapped into the seat. Once the ride started, we were suddenly thrown outward and jerked upward at the same time. My stomach was left behind like on a fast elevator." That, in a nutshell, describes the experiences of patients after a crisis: 1) the feeling of being strapped in, 2) the feeling of being pushed out, and 3) the feeling of being pulled up. In other words, there are three identifiable stages: in, out, and up. Let's begin with "in."

Implosive Inside

What Freud and Jung uncovered in the Victorian era has now openly manifested itself in our modern world. There is some dark chasm underneath the surface of our lives where the real person lives, in the shadowy world of the subconscious and dreams. All the passions of life reside here, those used for both constructive and destructive purposes. According to Straus, the yearly incidence of abusive acts within the population has a ratio of 4 out of every 100 persons in America (Gelles, 1985:356). These incidents take place in a variety of settings; many occur in the home: child abuse, couple violence, and abuse of the elderly. What concerns us is not so much the accuracy of these estimates, but the question of why does it occur in the first place? Health professionals see the results of these statistics on a regular basis in their offices and in the emergency rooms across this land.

Sociologists have identified several major characteristics associated with aspects of domestic violence. Gelles summarized social factors associated with this type of violence:

> 1) An intergenerational dynamic following a predictable cycle.
> 2) Low socioeconomic status and inadequate resources.

3) High stress in social and structural relations.
4) Social isolation with little community involvement.
5) Low self-esteem and feelings of inadequacy.
6) Personality problems with evidence of
    psychopathology.

Such approaches and questions lead to a variety of explanations; all of which are necessary if we are to understand the dynamics of loss and to ultimately learn to control our reactions. The process or impact of emotions cannot be directed, however, unless we first find an appropriate model which can serve as a diagnostic tool for our own evaluation. But the kind of model which simply clarifies is lacking. And as long as we are unclear about our reactions, there is less likelihood of diverting our emotions. While Denzin does produce two models, both are rather theoretical in nature. What I am proposing is the practical application of these modern insights in a useful model on emotive behavior (Figure 5-2).

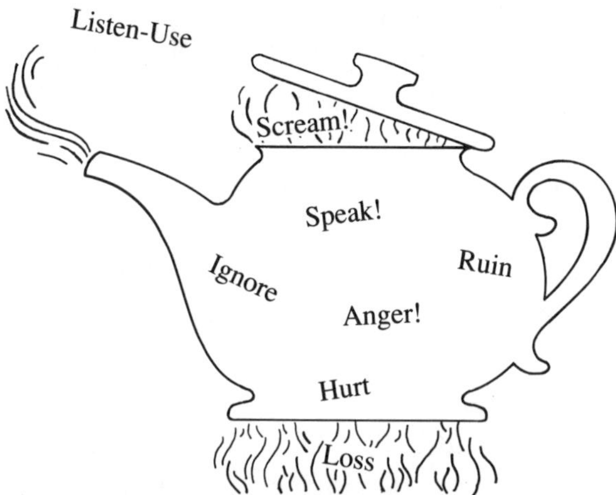

Figure 5-2. Steaming-Pot Emotions.

It was Freud who popularized the term "catharsis" to describe the need for a release of unconscious tension built up because of stress. While Freud defined emotions as physical in nature, Scheff (1979) identifies four basic types of stress emotions and their respective observable patterns: grief— weeping; fear— shivering; anger— laughter; and boredom —storming. Once emotions build up, like steam in a pot, there will eventually be release, either spontaneous or cathartic. Spontaneous discharge is uncontrollable; cartharsis can occur either by recall or reevaluation with a counselor as a guide. Both approaches, however, result in a drastic emotional change: from distress to discharge, and the reestablishment of an equilibrium.

This overview points to the importance of discipline orientation as a basis for comparisons. One issue still debated is whether emotions depend upon this stream of existential life encounters (Lacan) or whether emotions emerge only from physical sources. Following in the tradition of William James, Scheff sees emotions as being involuntary responses produced by the body under stress. Thus anything which releases these tensions (catharsis) contributes to healing and recovery.

Slaby and Glicksman (1985:184) discovered some interesting reactions of terminally ill patients. Among other observations, they noted that life-threatening illness caused their patients to become much more sensitive to their own bodily functions. They therefore believe that giving accurate information about a condition to patients is crucial to the physical and emotional well-being of the patient. In fact, this response is normal for children and occupies their whole attention. It is only as adults that we learn to disregard our bodily functions as we pursue other goals and interests. Illness, especially a terminal illness, reverses this process as the adult patient once again focuses upon his body.

This body sensitivity finds expression in several ways. People become very attentive to words they hear from doctors or friends. A colleague came down with a serious illness on his travels in Germany. While he could not understand much that was being said in German, he understood, or thought he did, "two years." This misinterpretation of the seriousness of his illness caused him a great deal of depression and grief. Only later did he learn that this was a misinterpretation. Under these circumstances, a patient copes better when words are encouraging and supportive.

The importance of social interaction can not be underestimated. Luchterhand (1971) found that the indiscriminate violence of natural disasters produces less permanent emotional damage than the discriminate punishment inflicted by another human being. Besides a secure social network of family and friends, a natural disaster can have mitigating factors based on scope, speed, duration, and preparedness.

Introspective analysis occurs throughout our lives. Rarely do we find such intensity, however, as in our encounter with a loss. It is during this time that we examine, as never before, just how we think and feel about our circumstances in life. Because we are often confused, we start at the most logical place, our feelings and thoughts.

Woodson observes that all intervention strategies in hospice care "acknowledge that in any organic disease or dysfunction there is always an emotional pain component operating in concert with, or in opposition to, pain associated with terminal disease" (1979:329). In such circumstances, pain and its relief are most important, but they must be balanced with care that requires special understanding of the implosion taking place within the patient, and that demands a "skillful blending of both the art of knowing how to listen with the third ear to the patient in pain and the science of seeing with the third eye what his or her needs are" (Woodson, 1979:326).

Explosive Outside

The implosion within produces an explosion without. This is a normal response to the loss of control over one's life. It can become abnormal, depending on the person. Reactions such as anxiety, depression, and agitation are most common. What seems to come forth first are unresolved conflicts (Salby and Glicksman, 1985:185).

Under these circumstances, the tensions of earlier periods come bursting forth, since our past experience determines much in how we respond to present circumstances. This is why those already experiencing some problems exhibit extreme cases of emotional trauma. Those earlier difficulties find current expression in strong feelings of unworthiness, bitterness, and hopelessness.

We will more easily solve the emotional difficulties associated with loss or illness when we integrate our strategies in health care with those that others have found important in clinical research. How people respond emotionally to the crisis of terminal illness has been documented by Woodson. He uses the idea of social pain to understand the sudden bursts of emotions toward others and ourselves. Using examples from hospices, Woodson lists several ways that this explosion may be exhibited:

1) People resent the inhumanity found in social life, both historically and contemporarily. This emotional reaction may be mild or rather intense in its manifestation.
2) People often feel uneasy about interpersonal relationships which, in the case of the dying, often become stressful.
3) People need emotional release through the process of anticipatory grief, grief, grief work, and bereavement. All of these needs require time and cannot be rushed.
4) In the case of terminal illness, people need to discuss certain legal requirements, family matters, and other unfinished business.
5) People must learn to say good-bye to what is lost, during this time in their lives (Woodson,1979:330-331).

Groups can help or harm the individual in problem solving matters. They may guide the individual to see some issues not previously considered, but because of personal preferences or life styles, this can become unacceptable. With counsel comes much information about options and items to salvage, but the ultimate decision is really up to the individual. That is the person who will be most affected by any decisions made. Outside of our lives, we find friends and enemies, those that are close and those that are distant; we talk and we listen; we like people and we hate people; we touch some and avoid others.

As Denzin says, "violence enacted (lived out) through emotions is a subjective, interactive process that places the person (the family members) in the presence of another"(1984:171). But such acts, directed outward, have certain requirements:

1) inversion of every attitude and emotion
2) connection of violent behavior with the victim
3) explanation for what happens
4) interaction with people in a social context

Violence follows when social constraints no longer work, and anyone is susceptible to taking violent action under those conditions. Violent emotions are sometimes contradictory when one person, for example, places the victim in a double bind; simultaneously harming the person while telling them that they love him or her. The abuse may not always be physical; it can be emotional. In those cases the mixed messages naturally are hard to decipher; the violence may be done in jest, but with violent consequences. These actions are clearly dissogenic.

Transplosive Anotherside

Nobody knows the boundaries of life better than those who go up to the edges and manage somehow to return from near disaster. It really does not matter how they got to the brink of disaster so much as what happens next. In English, as in other languages, there is a term for this: *brinkmanship*. These individuals push a dangerous situation to the limits before returning. Beyond that limit, there is no return. If the medical help is not enough when such a person has gone over the edge, the emotions shift toward a higher being or purpose for life. This is much like the professional actor who can find himself at times unable to differentiate reality from fiction. Sometimes the lines aren't all that clearly defined.

Changes in a patient's outlook usually occur in direct proportion to the disruptive nature of events. "Transplosive anotherside" refers to the emotional disruptions which tend to shatter people's basic assumptions and structures of meaning. These emotional dynamics are useful in understanding not only how people make choices, but also how they interpret consequences. Rapid or drastic changes produce constructive and destructive emotions which eventually influence how patients view the world and their place in it. Basic to this process are the beliefs which people hold, beliefs which significantly influence how one views the world. Jacobson (1986:251) says that assumptions, structures of meaning, and beliefs "...refer to the significance, meaning, and implications that an event or demand has for the individual's well-being."

The term "transplosive anotherside" refers to those basic emotions which determine one's outlook on life, such as religious beliefs, for example. People find comfort and express emotional relief with these beliefs, and an understanding of them should contribute to the quality of health care. This is not the place for a detailed analysis of the relationship between particular beliefs and medical treatment. Nor are these ideas presented to reduce the importance of specific beliefs. Our purpose is to examine how patients' beliefs influence their behavior, and to use that information to improve the quality of health care. Medical technology and health care professionals are limited in what can be done for some patients. Elizabeth Kubler Ross explored the full implications of this limitation and found that during those difficult periods of medical science limitations, patients often seek assistance from others. The patient uses "emotional radar" to probe toward some type of "transplosive anotherside." And that may take several forms, depending upon the particular community from which the person has come. Lovinger (1984:83-84) summarized several of these forms of religion:

1) Beliefs and ritual about a divine being
2) Ethical standards of social relations
3) The basis for solving internal and external conflicts
4) A mechanism for social integration and restoration
5) Allows for inconsistencies of assumed powers
6) Gives order and meaning to the world

It may be a personal philosophy, family tradition, or a religious belief. But whatever form these expressions take, they often guide ethical and moral behavior in everyday experiences. Since they are important practices and beliefs to the person when well, they will also prove to be important to that same person when he or she is sick.

We can study some examples of what form these expressions of oneness with the source of all life may take. Among the Alaskan Indians, a terminally ill person makes specific plans about their departure, including their final death rituals. To not take part would be most dishonorable. There is comfort in praying and singing to God, as well as talking and listening to family and friends (Woodson, 1979:331).

In the Jewish, Hindu, Buddhist, or Christian tradition, these fundamental expressions of unity with all (both family and God) give comfort and hope to the emotionally distraught. Whatever form these expression take, they "must be recognized as such and treated appropriately by the appropriate person" (Woodson, 1979:333). Pastors, rabbis, and priests "are highly skilled listeners, especially in those times of profound spiritual silence"(1979:333).

Profound silence causes most of us to direct our emotions outward, toward the unity of life itself. We are forced toward silence because there is solace in those moments. Sennett has listed silence as one way toward which our emotions are directed. Most writings on stress management recognize the importance of meditation. But often we only look up when we have to. We are too busy to consider the ultimate question of "Why?" Such questions aren't considered important during most of life. Only when we experience loss do we ask "Why?"

Sometimes we fondly remember the emotional sense of awe; other times we want to forget. Existentially, our feelings are mixed: we believe and then we doubt; we pray and then we curse; we submit and then we resist. There is the anticipation of something better, and the dread of something worse. Ultimately, each of us knows that we will give in and then give up; then we will make our peace before parting from this life. Even when on the brink of disaster, life must be lived right up until one dies. From interviews of 115 people, Veninga (1985:271-281) discovered some important lessons from those living through the emotional trauma of such experiences.

    1) To live for the moment, since that is all you can be
       assured of.
    2) To complete all unfinished business before it is too late.
    3) To celebrate life as long as you can.
    4) To love, for nothing can destroy fear but love alone.

Rather than ignoring other sources of power around us, it is our failure to utilize them that is the greater danger. Kennison (1987) believes that a holistic approach to patient care should tap this health resource. Although there are different dimensions of faith, people derive strength from their beliefs. During health crises, "some doubt the therapeutic affect of faith. There are still others who acknowledge faith as a facilitator of health" (Kennison, 1987:30). So losses might give rise to longings for new understandings where people rediscover new responses to a power which overcomes their frailties and weaknesses, to a power not unsympathetic to their suffering and deepest longings. Cousins describes that power resident in the human mind and body (1976), while

Muggeridge defines that power in historic Christian terms: "As man alone, Jesus could not have saved us; as God alone, he would not; Incarnate, he could and did." Gaylin recognizes that power in the next generation. That is why the death of a child takes on a different dimension: "For those of us who have no religion at all, the loss of the child is the loss of the only immortality we recognize—the continuation of our genes through our children" (Gaylin, 1986:174). That power is also social when patients trust those in the medical professions to do the impossible. What happens when these same professionals lose faith in their abilities is predictable. Because terminal cancer victims might "perceive that the nurses and other health care professionals no longer trust in a cure, a primary source of strength and hope withers. In contrast, it is possible to energize these same clients by discovering and fostering whatever store of faith they wish to exhibit" (Kennison, 1987:30).

Summary and Conclusions

In the solitude of a moment of loss and grief, patients may think they are alone with their private thoughts, but they are not. Even though it appears that they stand alone, isolated from the fast-paced tempo of life, they stand where others have stood before and where all will one day stand. This peculiar mood is common to all: to believe something about ourselves which in reality is quite the opposite from that which in fact exists. The common vulnerability that we all experience is the social quality that demonstrates the solidarity of the human race.

What we eventually come to realize is the universal experience of emotional grief that follows personal or collective losses. It is through this type of experience that we can identify with others. For to be human is to experience loss, pain, and tears. When we discover this vital connection between life and loss, we then see how emotions exist only in opposition to community life. "Emotional attachments ... require a social presence, a provisional order, and even a daily routine" (Unger 1986:63). Because of our common experiences in illness and loss, we can sympathize with others in a detached manner. But sympathy involves more than that. "Sympathy includes a recognition of comic incongruity: the incongruity between the state that someone is in, whether of weakness and suffering or strength and elation, and the deeper conditions of selfhood that combine embodiment and finitude with a longing for the unconditional" (Unger,1986:235).

Our lives then depend upon society, but what happens when that society is itself experiencing rather tumultuous changes? And what happens when destructive emotions outweigh the constructive ones? We have explored the implications of these issues in the previous two chapters, and we have discussed how emotive analysis and therapies might work together in identifying emotional dynamics.

Yet no matter what the suggestions about how to prepare patients for crisis or how to work with patients during or after crisis, one fact remains obvious. When recipients have learned to respect their emotions more than their physical health, they shall respect their physical health better than they do now. Conversely, as they learn to respect the physical at the expense of the emotional, they move toward a condition in which they respect neither. When put in proper perspective, the parts are not negated as supposed, but enhanced. This fact will be demonstrated with a discussion of emotive analysis and therapy in the following chapter.

Chapter 6

Emotive Analysis and Therapy

Behavioral scientists in the Soviet Union give less attention to "emotions and feelings" than to "thinking and learning." Comparing the incidence of articles by research topic, Cacioppo and Petty (1983) found that the greatest difference was on the topic of emotions. Western social scientists regularly explore factors associated with emotions; the significance of an experience for recall is one example. "Flashbulb memories" refers to the mental ability of people to recall detailed information. Some events—assassinations, accidents, disappointments—not only contain intense emotions, but they also imprint detailed information for long periods of time (Brown:1986:269-281). Not surprisingly, the Soviet researchers follow the Pavlovian tradition when studying emotions and a topic such as flashbulb memories.

In 1914, Pavlov experimented on the nervous centers of animals. He studied the conditioned responses of dogs to bell sounds and the effects on body functions. Pavlov later applied his lab procedures to the nervous system of humans. Although he was dealing with a more complex system containing inborn reflexes, conditioned reflexes, and language, Pavlov did not give much attention to the sociopsychological aspects of emotions. Researchers in the Pavlovian tradition see stressful activities as precipitating in the physiological mechanisms and as being regulated by the cerebral cortex (brain) at both the somatic and autonomic levels. Soviet scientists occasionally study somatovisceral factors. In one such study of the subjective experiences of parachutists, heart and respiration rates (a function of lung ventilation) were measured just before the critical moment when the parachutists jump from the plane. Surprisingly, experienced jumpers registered higher heart and ventilation (somatovisceral) rates than inexperienced jumpers. Their past experience of jumps and their anticipation of the impending jump (subjective factor) affected their rates. Not knowing what to expect protects inexperienced jumpers. Evidently, subject anticipation makes the difference. Soviets rarely analyzed the subjective, while Americans frequently study subjective factors which elicit these patterns of emotions. This approach is characterized, for example, by studies which might concentrate on such factors as facial expressions, meanings attributed to those expressions, and the perceptions people hold. Hedin and Haas (1984:959) emphasized the importance of subjective factors in their study dealing with the adaptations of Vietnam veterans: "what our findings appear to suggest is the importance of looking more closely at perceptual and adaptive factors, rather than simply at objective aspects of the combat experience in seeking to explain why some veterans have been more severely distressed after their return from Vietnam, while others have not." Another example of such a study of subjective factors is the study on postservice mortality by the Centers for Disease Control (1987:795): "if Vietnam veterans tended to have an inherent predisposition to traumatic events, it might be expected to manifest itself in increased mortality from such causes throughout the period of observation, not just in the first few years, as observed here."

Whether studying individuals as parachutists, in combat, or as patients in hospitals, these studies all identify the intrasubjective dimensions of stress. Just as seasoned veterans know what the next jump means, so do cancer victims who anticipate the next painful treatment. Both the experienced and inexperienced groups respond quite similarly; both show signs of stress, increased heart rates, respiration rates, and lung ventilation; but for different reasons.

Since health care varies with the physiological and emotional responses of patients, intrasubjective perceptions are important. Professionals may be able to stabilize patients by explaining physiological changes and by recognizing subjective feelings.

Sensitive care and aftercare recognizes intrasubjective responses in patients. Early diagnosis of cancer increases chances of survival; Broadwell (1987) studied some of the issues around cancer diagnosis and treatment. What he discovered about emotions is full of meaning for health care workers. Professionals who sensitively impart information minimize the anxiety, if not the intensity, of bodily pain. The fact is that sympathetic and sensitive people predict the beginnings of illness more often than those less inclined. These experiences, according to Broadwell, don't fit current models of emotions—fearful, disease disabilities. The sensitive patients have functional dynamic abilities. They have the same information as others, but they use it differently. Sensitive people process their bodily information, monitor bodily feedback, and make appropriate adjustments. They are able to change their behavior in illness or crisis. Their emotive analysis leads to their therapy.

A New Perspective

Scientists cautiously form and test ideas about their subjects. Their objective is to mirror reality, not to construct it. To mirror is to "think of science as a concrescence, a growing together of variable, interacting, mutually reinforcing factors, contributing to a development organic in character" (Black, 1954:23). Some scientists use the analogy of a fishing net as an imaginative, dialectic tool to test their ideas. Whatever the metaphor, "growing together" or "sewing a net," scientists decipher hidden meaning, interpret symbols and perceptions of people, and make visible their sources. Imagination of this sort guided Einstein, beyond either the facts-to-concepts (induction) or the concepts-to-facts (deduction), as he formulated images of energy.

When scientific ideas don't seem to mirror reality, people invent metaphors. It is commonly recognized "that organizations are not organized to the extent that the metaphor 'organization' suggests they should be; this provides an impetus for their conceptualization in other's terms, e.g., as political systems, garbage cans, psychic prisons, or whatever" (Morgan, 1983:603;1986). The observations are not devoid of meaning, although the metaphors to explain organizations are. What is debated about metaphors is whether or not, as subjective mirrors of organizations, they have significance for practitioners who use these formulations to treat diseases and people. Scientists sometimes don't distinguish between the metaphorical and the literal. This is how humans engage, organize, and understand their world. Equal weight is given to both types of language because work—perception, language, memory, knowledge—takes place as structured experience. Those who do make a distinction prefer a precise language which fits the scientific models of operational definitions, hypothesis testing, and theory development. It is the metaphor, not the literal approach, that characterizes our proposed new perspective.

In the writings of some, crisis is neglected; Erik Erikson emphasizes it in his work. Erikson evaluated human life and experiences through homeostatic and interactive lenses. In the eight stages of life, people face a series of psychosocial crises. *Each crisis, regardless of the particular stage, is resolved only through significant relations with others.* The crisis of young adults involves polar extremes of intimacy or isolation. Only as young adults establish friends and work together can they pass through crisis. To not do so is to risk isolation. To engage friends is to love—"that elusive and yet all-pervasive power of cultural and personal style which binds into a 'way of life' the affiliations of competition and cooperation, procreation and production. The problem is one of transferring the experience of being cared for in a parental setting to an adult affiliation, actively chosen and cultivated, as a mutual concern within a new generation" (Schlein, 1987:607).

Similarly, the purpose for an emotive analysis and therapy is to provide yet another perspective from which to view the emotional responses of those needing quality health care. Serendipitous insights about human emotions may come from a different view of the ordinary. To ensure this, Erickson always used symptoms established in interpersonal relations as a starting place for prescribing therapy. Then he tried to reconstitute, not eliminate, symptoms. So "treatment needs to concentrate more on altering the patient's current and future behaviors than on understanding and communicating the extent to which past events have lead to the patient's present maladjustments" (Seltzer, 1986:101). It is a "here and now" perspective. New insights into the causes of illness or responses may come from the patients themselves. This happens only as providers help to gain an understanding of symptoms. Revising models not only multiples the possibilities of analyses, but more importantly, it increases the alternatives for therapy. However, a course of action other than those currently used is possible only if the proposed approach is reliable and valid.

To ensure quality health care is to assume the need for a perspective on functional dynamic abilities, not fearful diseased disabilities. Whether as a nurse, mental health specialist, social worker, or psychiatrist, therapy for those injured or ill tests new insights about fluctuating patterns of emotions. How does the social context of emotions apply to the dazed and bewildered feelings immediately following an accident? And how are these connections between emotions and interaction to be made? In a world where losses abound, construed models about the cause-effect relationship of losses also abound. The National Institute of Mental Health recently published several models representing the cause-effect chain of events leading up to and following emotional crises.

As important as causal models are for understanding prevention and treatment of stress, this chapter gives priority not just to the physical causes, but also to the emotions they produce. Symptoms of emotional distress vary more than physical symptoms. Since health care providers naturally emphasize the physiological responses, *an appropriate model should encompass both the institutional, or community settings, and the quality care necessary to buffer these expanding emotions*. The providers, not the equipment, make the difference when service is tailored to health recipients. Yet the process must be easily understood and practically administered if the emotive analysis and therapy are to work.

Sensitivity to the patient's physical and emotional needs forms the partnership which encourages quality care appropriate to the occasion. It's like adding rooms to a house to allow for an expanding family of emotions. New babies crowd a small house; covert feelings and overt behavior crowd the emotional structure of the patient, unless providers add extra rooms for expanding emotions. For terminally ill cancer patients, it is usually easier to die at home in the security of one's family than in an isolated ward surrounded by a medical team. As Elizabeth Kobler Ross said: "Let a person live right up until the time they die." The familiar though often unrecognized social patterns may provide support and security that is extremely valuable during a terminal illness.

Without emotional support, the patient is neither able to interpret the intruders of loss nor preserve the emotional energy necessary to overcome them. For in addition to dealing with intruders (loss in all forms), the patients must also allay their fears and assuage the resentment that those insidious intruders bring. In these cases, without the support of sympathetic others, there are no extra rooms for patients to put their emotional baggage. Conversely, sympathy comes from those who, though not having exactly the same type of disease, have similar emotional distress. It can be argued that few of us have not previously encountered some fears. These prototype experiences become doors of sympathy through which people walk. Even health care workers, on some occasions, symbolically become gates for their patients when these patients are hopelessly lost in the chaos of disruptions and stress. In all branches of science, models guide advances. But in the case of emotional distress, most models are inappropriate. One element eludes researchers; and that is the very quality by which people are people. In the description of people, the sensitive can detect incongruity. But providers who understand people recognize this neglected dimension.

The Statue of Liberty

To perceive how people perceive emotions is to include the aesthetic and poetic—the intuition of clients and the sentiments of society. The meaning of emotions is automatically computed from out of that; it is socially constructed in the patterns of interaction. From these come belonging and identity, as evidenced by opinion polls and user surveys. These cohesive boundaries are distinctive and notable, yet destructive in dissogenic families. Crucial issues in troubled families revolve around the communication of feelings. "Many people who have self-image problems and difficulty with intimate relationships believe, rightly or wrongly, that their parents do not love them. Promoting communication of such feelings can therefore be an important part of the treatment of some families" (Barker, 1985:142). Establishing communication can, however, unleash raw emotions that can cause problems. Sometimes a story objectifies tensions and diverts them away from specific people, allowing for the establishment of more communication with less emotional upset. By using stories, people also understand their own social definitions of situations, and in a nonthreatening way they can see how people fit together. That is why many therapists recommend the ancient method of story-telling.

Most metaphors and stories in a culture do have a message. The story of Humpty Dumpty, for example, warns us to "be careful what you do because sometimes even the experts can't repair the damage resulting from ill-judged acts" (Barker, 1987:10). A story gives new insights into old problems in two unique ways: "It involves a reframing of an experience, and it offers a view of an incident from a later point in time. These two processes—reframing and considering how things appear when looked back upon later—can help clients deal with certain kinds of emotional problems" (Barker, 1985:110). Everyone is interested in how "to turn liabilities into assets by pointing out different aspects of a situation or person. When one views problems as also being attempted solutions, one works to create new solutions to replace symptomatic attempts to achieve personal or family goals" (L'Abate, et al., 1986:61). L'Abate argues for two facets of therapy; one is aesthetic and emphasizes "the importance of subjective, phenomenological experience, and the supremacy of emotions in the functionality or dysfunctionality of family"; the other emphasizes "the importance of an objective methodology and substantive expertise to obtain changes in clinical families" (L'Abate,1986:6-7). The former is style, an "aesthetic, human quality"; the latter is method, "the pragmatic quality of the therapist's professional preparation and competence, which include repeatable types of intervention" (L'Abate,1986:7).

Baker recommends both the style and method of story-telling. Depressed people, for instance, readily identify with the the wilderness wonderings of the Hebrews, or other struggling travelers (1985:125). What illustrates hopeful struggle better than the Statue of Liberty, a symbol of freedom to those subject to oppression. Known to immigrants as the Isle of Tears, they ironically associated Ellis Island with Liberty. "If Liberty symbolized the aspirations, ideals, and dreams of immigrants, Ellis Island would come to represent the harsh realities and ordeals they would have to endure before they and their children would share in America's blessings" (Shapiro, 1986:6).

No modern monument is comparable. Historically, people have dedicated monuments to military victory, to those who gave their lives, or to some prominent leader. This monument, however, was the idea of a French law professor (Edouard de Laboulaye) who was known for his expertise on the U.S. Constitution. He asked the sculptor Frederic-Auguste Bartholdi to design Liberty as the triumph of independence over repression.

Health professionals symbolically "see" their patients through models such as Liberty. This section will explain the value of this visual symbol. More than embellishment, this symbol is constitutive in nature. The analogy of Liberty conveys important insights about three categories of human emotions—motivation, feeling, and affection. The anthropologist Wagner (1986) used a similar approach—analogy and its holography of meaning—to show the interrelation between natural kinship units among the Daribi in New Guinea. Similarly, the analogy of Liberty is symbolically significant beyond just the recognition of three categories of emotions. This symbolism should be useful in analyzing and responding to emotions. Each of these purposes is presented below in separate sections dealing with analysis and therapy.

Analyzing Social Emotions

Analyzing emotions is essential to coping with them. Some of the material on sociological descriptions in Chapter 4 is integrated into the present discussion via an analogical approach. The analogical model of a triangle is shown in Figure 6-1. That basic model has six identifiers: three angles and three legs. Each is an important concept for analyzing social emotions.

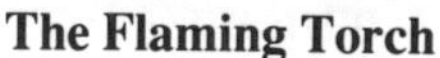

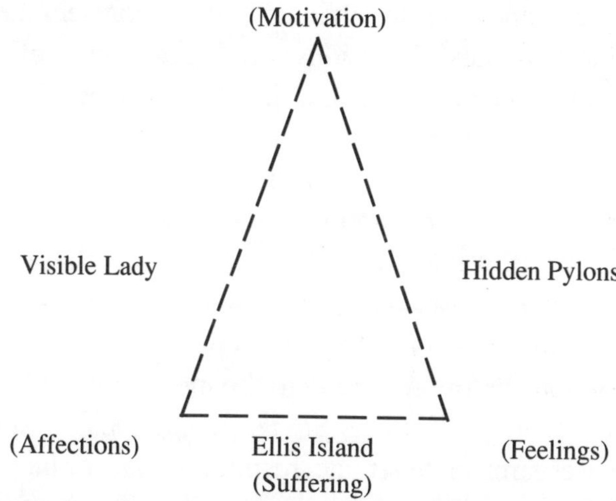

Figure 6-1. An Analogy of Emotions.

After loss, people's emotions are pulled away immediately and uncontrollably from the motivation of normal activities. These emotions go downward, toward Ellis Island (Figure 6-1), where feelings (inwardly directed emotions) and affections (outwardly oriented emotions) cause intense suffering. This imbalance of emotions leads to depression and even compulsiveness. The compulsiveness may turn towards violence, alcohol, and drugs. The configuration of past and present social influences comes into prominence: a minor family accident may overwhelm some; a major disequilibrium may sensitize others. Some groups live on the brink of disaster, so any slight disruptions triggers violent emotions. *Others live closely linked together so that they buffer each other during times of disruption, allowing members to go beyond their individual capacities.* Those providers who understand the sociology of emotions will improve their diagnostic skills and their ability to use therapy more effectively.

Emotions are a function of time—present, future, and past—and both positive and negative experiences affect people's emotions (see Figure 6-1). The labels for the two lower legs in figure 6-1 are "Visible Lady" and "Hidden Pylons;" they represent the visible and invisible dynamics of emotions as an energy source of life. That is why emotions can explode in a time of loss (see Figure 4-1 if needed). After the emotional explosion, the remains fall onto Ellis Island. It is after a loss or illness that health care recipients begin to cope with uncontrollable emotions, emotions labelled "Feelings," and "Affection" (lower angles in Figure 6-1). Since these two terms refer to specific emotional categories, since both terms are central to this discussion, and since they encompass earlier material, note their distinctions before returning to the metaphor of Liberty.

The term "feelings" reflects Soviet perceptions on autonomic responses. Research on heart rate, respiration rate, or lung ventilation has demonstrated the physiological effect of stressful experiences. Soviet researchers have observed and measured emotions with the instrumentation of modern science. Their American counterparts study the subjective effects of emotions mainly in three areas. Though not limited to these areas alone, Americans researchers observe facial expressions, meanings attributed to those expressions, and perceptions people hold of them. It is an emphasis on experienced emotions from embodied encounters; Americans emphasize live feelings that affect mortality. Both types of objective and subjective research reflect how patients process bodily information.

In the cycle of emotional response, feelings refer to accompanying reactions for each of these phases of a severe loss or illness: shock (numbness, disbelief), disorganization (despair, fear, franticness), searching (yearning, weeping, restlessness), and grief (fatigue, depression). The absence of initial feelings usually gives way to denial, despair, and fear. It is as if the shock temporarily numbed the senses and the emotional impact is silently endured as mourning and grief. Only later are some of these embodied feelings manifested, and the invisible feelings become obvious. The provider sees this manifestation in such forms as weeping, restlessness, fatigue, and depression. For the most part, these emotions are inwardly directed toward the self, even though the experience may involve someone or something outside of the self. In other words, there are initially few words which express these deep feelings of grief after a loss or illness.

The feelings go not go away, however. Feelings are involuntary and invisible responses to everyday experiences. As people continue to experience losses—health, independence, self-sufficiency, job, family—their emotions are continually directed toward the "world of emotions." While this emotional world differs from the everyday world, they are nevertheless interrelated. Stress is associated with emotions and crisis. Patients cope with a variety of emotions after crises: shock, numbness, denial, disbelief, anguish, sorrow, disorganization, anxiety, anger, frustration, resentment, franticness, searching, ambivalence, jealousy, yearning, weeping, restlessness, grief, fatigue, exhaustion, vulnerability, insecurity, uncertainty, guilt, shame, helplessness, hopelessness, confusion, and depression. Words are not really capable of describing what is happening within the individual; words are abstractions which pull people away from their experiences and emotions. Nevertheless, these categories do serve a purpose. They provide a framework for analyzing emotions and rendering treatment; but only people bearing the pain of distress know what the true meaning of these words is.

In contrast to "feelings," "affections" are those feelings emerging from interaction in a social context. Glaser and Strauss use the term "awareness context," while Mead writes about the concept of "sociality" (Denzin, 1984:131). The self is identified with something or someone emotionally. As a concept, affection includes all aspects of emotions, even the need for prolonged recovery. In a classic 1944 study on grief, Erich Lindemann discussed the processes of emotional emancipation, withdrawal, and reinvestment in new relationships (Rando,1986:3). Current research indicates that *interpersonal affections act as emotional buffers, but only as people provide emotional support.* Even with the best emotional and social support, everyone still goes through some cycle of emotions during grief. That cycle includes: guilt, shame (letting go), anger, helplessness, hopelessness, and confusion (separation). Attention to these affections affects patients and their current status of emotions.

While feelings are inwardly directed, the affections are outwardly directed toward someone or something. However, in both cases their manifestations may become evident through mourning, crying, and grieving. The distinction is in terms of focus, not in manifest behavior, but the distinction between feelings and affections is useful in a nonsociological approach where social and interactive factors are easily overlooked.

The expression of feelings must be allowed to flow following the profound emotional experiences of tragedy or crisis. People express those feelings with metaphors like "my stomach's in knots," or "its full of butterflies," or "I'm shaking like a leaf." The intense feelings that follow a health crisis should be released as they expand. One way is by crying: "Instinctively, I knew that I had to pay attention to my feelings....I also knew instinctively that this would take time...I felt deeply and I cried. I believe to this day that it was the healthiest way to mourn"(Weizman and Kamm,1986:73). Anger and guilt can still be evident. People start to think about what happened, what might have happened, what should have happened—all of these thoughts move the person to higher forms of mental anguish and a prescribed moral order in a sociological sense. Thus, we can say that while initial emotions are body centered and body felt through the senses, later reflections move toward higher levels of emotional processing. That is where a sociological understanding of traditions, customs, and history becomes important.

Patients direct their emotional attention away from normal activities, downward toward Ellis Island where feelings (inwardly directed emotions) and affections (outwardly oriented emotions) can disrupt emotional health. Some group relations push people to the brink of disaster; others provide a buffer, allowing them to go beyond their individual capacities. Consequently, as these two lower emotional needs are met, the recovering individual can better cope, moving upward from mourning toward health motivation (the top angle on Figure 6-1).

As time in mourning passes, the provider eventually needs to consider the patient's need for reorienting, designated by the term "motivation." For once the person has bottomed out, he or she needs to enter the recovery phases: resolution (relief, peace), and reintegration (acceptance of loss and positive actions). This third top angle (Figure 6-1) suggests that most patients struggle for a desire (motivation) to carry on after illness. Motivation connotes carrying on after crisis, planning for the future. It also affects how patients reorganize themselves for the future, how they assume new roles and responsibilities, and how they network with others in the aftermath. In some instances, and with some people, this is more difficult to accomplish than at other times or with other people. In any case, emotional energy must be be properly channelled toward some beginning again. Health professionals can serve as the initial catalysts for such positive action. Their encouragement, in whatever form, affects the whole process of recovery and reintegration into social life.

Health professionals are aware that there are private and public dimensions in patients' lives. The fact that some aspects of a patient's life are private (not seen or immediately known to health professionals) does not suggest that they are useless. Those inside attitudes, values, and dreams may well be more of a motivating factor than the visible ones. Yet private feelings and affections are not what is seen; it is the public self that we display to the care givers around us.

The analogy of Liberty has visible and invisible elements reflecting that duality. Providers see only the outside, what is publicly known, but there is an intrinsic connection between what is outside and what is inside. Physical injuries affect how people feel about themselves, especially if that inner structure is already weakened. But like Liberty, people sometimes need overhauling, both at the inner level (invisible) and the outer level (visible). That's what sickness is all about—repairing those parts that need fixing.

We can use this analogy to assess patients. Starting with patients (Figure 6-1 at the bottom), note that both emotional categories (feelings—lower right and affections—lower left) are joined by the base line "Ellis Island" (suffering). We can sum up the lessons of the analogy of Liberty in Figure 6-1 as follows:

1) Illness and any kind of loss impacts a patient's emotions. As a result, people are emotionally dragged downward. Because of this downward pattern, motivation comes only after a struggle to get well or recover.

2) All three of these emotions (feelings, affections, motivation) are connected to both the visible and invisible aspects of patients'

lives. Some of these are observable to health care professionals, and others are private matters; often, they are unexpressed and inexpressible. However they are defined, recognized, or expressed, they are the energy source which propels the patient forward. That is why when the flame goes out, despondency and thoughts of suicide may naturally follow.

3) Motivation is at the top of the triangle because it symbolizes the flaming torch of that emotional energy; and at this point, we're back where we started. Motivation depends upon the other structures of life: those visible and those invisible; those known and those unknown; those used and those not used. Thus, to be well means that emotional energy is constructively directed and securely connected with the other components of life. Under normal circumstance, there is more likely to be a unity and wholeness of purpose which constructively motivates the person than in times of sickness or upheaval.

Utilizing Emotive Therapy

The degree of patient motivation after loss depends upon the structures (beams and pylons) of their lives. Some of these "anchorage beams" and "load bearing steel" (hidden pylons) are below the surface of their lives. Other structures—the crown, face, body—remain more visible. In either case, health professionals render proper treatment so that patients can achieve maximum recovery. Their role as symbols of hope is analogous to that of "Liberty" herself.

The analogy of Liberty is also a vehicle for quality health care. Its language is consistent with that of the health professions. It is useful because it conveys some insights about emotions that other explanations do not. These insights are useful not only in the analysis, but also in the treatment that follows. The elements of this analogy are based on field observations reported by social scientists and recognized by health professionals. The analogy has both utility and validity as a type of health care analysis.

With these suggestions in mind (both the analysis and the

analogy), providers can visualize their utility in emotive therapy. This section extends the earlier ones; the triangle is used to examine what emotive therapy means to providers and patients. That, however, necessitates changes in labels, but not in the basic analogy of visible and invisible structures (Figure 6-2). In the earlier sections, the analysis was directed towords the patient; here it's focused on the partnership between the provider and the patient.

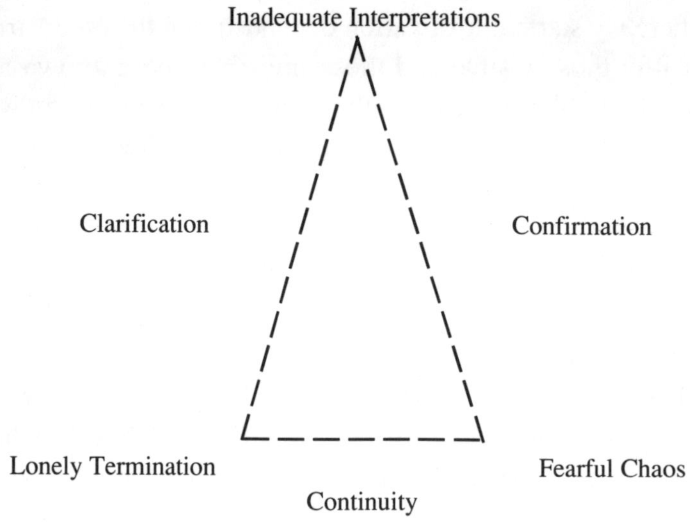

Figure 6-2. A Therapy for Action.

Before using this analogy, it might help to survey the changes and the rationale. In the earlier triangle (Figure 6-1) nothing was considered outside the basic arrangement of three legs and angles. That is not the case here. Figure 6-2 describes the patient's immediate emotional needs; then it prescribes what the provider does; and finally it promotes an understanding of the partnership. Taken in that order, changes describe emotional needs. The changes and additions to Figure 6-1 convey these differences."Feelings" are replaced with "fearful chaos"; "affections" replaced with "lonely termination"; and "motivation" with "inadequate interpretations."

These new terms are more than synonyms; they refer to the negative emotional dispositions often observed in patients. After a crisis, feelings often result in fearful chaos where patients are bewildered about what has happened, what is happening, and what will happen. It's a new experience, filled with pain, confusion, and disorientation.

Change also prescribes emotional needs. The analogy of Liberty is an externally constituted relationship; but it can also be an internally related one. The discussion previously was limited to the triangle's external features: one angle and only its relationship to those two immediate sides which formed it. Internal triangular changes also change the explanations. These internal changes are shown in Figure 6-2. For each of the three angles, visualize another line drawn across to the leg. Perpendicular lines are drawn from each of the three corners to the opposite side. These new lines sequence the internal relations, thereby implying the complexity of emotional responses. The lower right corner is connected with the leg labelled "clarification," the lower left corner with the leg labelled "confirmation," and the upper corner with the leg labelled "continuity."

Plato said that "when hope leaves, despondency begins." That is why interactions (clarification) give clarity to patients as they stop lamenting the past and focus on the future. Yet doubt persists without the encouragement from spouse, friends, or professionals who explore the feelings and goals of the afflicted (confirmation). Finally, the functional dynamic abilities of patients are actualized when they maximize their potential within the constraints of disease/treatment. That is why reality surveys should not destroy the will to continue (continuity) in spite of difficulties.

These triangular changes also highlight the patient's immediate emotional needs. That is why a change in the triangle implies changes in our thinking about the patient. Specifically, patients have complex emotional needs, needs which spell quality health care. They are listed below as metaphors:

1) A person with a traumatizing loss may feel like a paralyzed fly caught in a spider's web. This represents the line from "fearful chaos" diagonally across to "clarification."

2) It is often after a series of knockout losses that a patient sees about as clearly as a punch-drunk boxer. This represents the line from "lonely termination" across to "confirmation."

3) The loss syndrome and the despair of loneliness come after crisis. Emotionally, such people frantically search and hopelessly wait for what has been lost. They are much like a devoted dog who at first chases, then watches for, its master's departed car. This represents the line from "inadequate interpretation" across to "continuity."

What can the health care professional—nurse, physician, clinical psychologist, psychotherapist, psychiatric social worker, occupational therapist, educator, disaster worker—do in these cases? One answer is implicit in these internal changes: fearful chaos (clarification), lonely termination (confirmation), inadequate interpretations (continuity).

The exact nature of this therapy depends upon many factors, but this diagram allows health care professionals to see the issues involved. When the issues are clear they should be able to make better judgments about intervention and support. Figure 6-2 depicts "fearful chaos" opposite from "clarification." This aspect of the analogy suggests that human beings often need clarification of occurrences. It might be a provider's explanation about the effects of drugs, the nature of the illness, or the extent of an injury. To clarify what's ahead (to know what to expect) helps patients to dispel some of the uncertainty and fearful chaos. These activities of health care workers are usually taken for granted, but they are still important to patients.

The same procedure can be seen at work in the other angles. It all depends upon what the patient needs. The next angle is "lonely termination." If patients have little social support, then health care providers need to confirm the worth, dignity, and self respect of their patients. This appropriate action will in turn reduce the likelihood of loneliness. Clinical psychologists might give clients assignments to increase their interaction with others: making new friends, taking risks with others; these are typical assignments to help patients break the cycle of loneliness that can result from divorce, death, or severe illness.

The last angle of the triangle in Figure 6-2 is labelled "inadequate interpretations." An earlier model used the term "motivation," but here the term is "interpretation." The implication is that people who suffer emotional distress often need some interpretation about the meaning of life. Sometimes they lose their desire to live, and in those cases continuation of life (continuity) becomes a serious problem. What does life mean? What is its purpose? Where are we headed? Is there more to life than what we know or experience? All of these questions demand adequate interpretation. Who gives those interpretations? Many people do, including those with religious authority (priests, chaplains, ministers, rabbis). Words of encouragement help. Yes, this role is broader than medical training, but sensitive providers give quality health care.

A Case Study

What is it like to experience a life-changing loss? When Jean experienced her health crisis, it radically altered her life. Just before it happened, Jean remembered sitting out on her porch one night watching the stars. Little did she realize that one of those many mosquitoes she brushed away had infected her with encephalitis. When admitted to the hospital, Jean realized how sick she was. Under constant health care, providers told her about her serious condition. The worst experience came later as the disease spread throughout her body and to her brain. The full emotional impact of the disease was not realized until later. It was after hospitalization, brain swelling, surgery, unconsciousness, and blindness. Her grief continued into rehabilitation, when she began to see that life would not return to normal. That was when the real struggle began.

The emotions that she felt followed the pattern that we have seen for loss. First came the shock with disbelief that this was actually happening to her. She found herself in unfamiliar circumstances, extremely confused, fearful, anxious about the future, and rightly so, because death was imminent. In addition to other feelings, she also had to cope with her strong fear of death. To understand the exact relation between emotion, time, and the event of loss, it might help to analyze her emotions and then utilize the emotive therapy approach. Figure 6-1 shows how the social analysis works in times of crisis, and Figure 6-2 shows how therapy works. Emotional analysis and therapy can be contrasted in the case of Jean, her health care workers, and others described above. Here is a summary of what actually happened with the onset of her condition:

1) She immediately experienced uncontrollable reactions which promptly pulled her emotional energies away from the motivation of normal activities, downward toward Ellis Island, where her feelings and affections began to cause her intense suffering.

2) Once on the bottom, the visible and invisible dynamics of life exploded, with a variety of manifestations: shock (numbness, disbelief), disorganization (despair, fear, franticness), searching (yearning, weeping, restlessness), grief (fatigue, depression). The initial absence of feelings soon gave way to denial, despair, and fear.

3) Other reactions occurred later when she finally began to accept her blindness: letting go (guilt, shame), separation (anger, anxiety). While the first emotions (feelings) were inwardly directed, the next emotions (affections) were outwardly directed, toward others.

4) Once the life-threatening danger was over, she began to think about what had happened, what might have happened, and what should have happened; all of these thoughts moved her to higher forms of emotional anguish and a prescribed moral order. While initial emotions were body-centered and body-felt, through the senses, later reflections moved her toward higher levels emotional processing where she questioned her religious beliefs and reflected upon the injustices done to her.

5) Motivation was a problem, especially with her blindness. She did go through rehabilitation: resolution (relief, peace) and reintegration (acceptance of loss and positive actions), but she continued to struggle with a motivation for living until she began to find new sources of emotional energy. Health professionals supported her and served as catalysts for positive action, the challenge of recovery and reintegration into social life.

6) Health professionals clarified her physical condition so that she would accept the reality of blindness. They also consoled her with encouraging words and supportive behavior. Finally, they and others in her family listened as she revised her inadequate interpretations about what all of this meant.

Continuity and Change

Providers of health care begin with the patient's physical and emotional needs. The sociology of emotions provides creative insights about human emotions, but the partnership between provider and patient provides enough room to accomodate the expanding gap between the concrete experience of a crisis and its subsequent emotional upheaval. In other words, quality care bridges the gap between covert feelings and overt behavior.

Immediately following an accident, these two models (analysis and therapy) can help patients maintain emotional stability and begin their full recovery. Through proper implementation, patients begin to shift their dazed and bewildered emotions back toward a positive, planned motivational strategy. How are these connections to be made? The symptoms of emotional distress vary more than physical symptoms, but fortunately, providers now have checklists for understanding and designing the patient's recovery program. Patients who accurately interpret the intruders of loss may not be robbed of their emotional energy, energy which is necessary for them to become intrepid overcomers.

Quality health care requires accurate analyses of the patient's emotional state, which is a function of time and events. Both positive and negative experiences produce emotional energy. These surges of power have immediate, future, and long-term effects, and the patient must adjust to these changes. People can change their behavior if: 1) they want to and 2) if they are supported by others whom they respect. Since health professionals are highly respected, their support helps patients to stabilize both physically and emotionally.

After bottoming-out emotionally, patients begin their recovery of emotional health. Success depends on quality care and personal motivation. Patients need to regain what has been lost in the two "R Stages" of recovery: resolution (relief, peace) and reintegration (the acceptance of loss, subsequent positive actions). Each of these, however, depends upon other structures of life; those both visible and invisible, known and unknown, used and not used. The emotional energy comes from within the individual and their support groups, including the health professionals.

A time of loss is not an easy time for unity and wholeness of purpose, even with emotion buffers. Severe illness and crises leave their mark: emotional paralysis (the fly caught in the web); feelings of isolation and desertion (the punch-drunk boxer); and frantic searching for what is lost (the dog chasing after his owner's car). These metaphors suggest some action: 1) in the midst of fearful chaos; 2) after a period of lonely termination; and 3) at a time of inadequate interpretations (Figure 6-2). The therapeutic action discussed in this chapter relates to the quality care of providers who clarify emotional patterns, confirm personal worth, and encourage continuity of life.

Part III

Utilizing Emotional Intervention

Chapter 7

The Resource of Personal Encounters

The trauma of severely injured patients demands team interaction. Beginning at the accident site, rescuers have these priorities: 1) the preservation of life, 2) the avoidance of pain and complications, 3) evaluation for shock and the prevention of further injury. The health care team takes over from the rescuers and continues the patient care. The coordination is a complex interaction pattern centering around "who gives what to whom regarding which problems?" (House, 1981). Seeing the victims from an emotional angle is also important:

> When the severely injured patient has regained consciousness after the intensive care, he or she needs gentle, general care, with attention to psychological needs. Empathy, understanding, and adequate training are required of the personnel. Patients, especially if they are elderly, often wish for the comforting words of a clergyman. Such words may not only offer the patient the consolation of religion, but also may motivate him or her to cooperate with the team. From the very beginning, the patient should feel that the staff is not only concerned about the present medical situation, but also about him or her, as an individual with anxieties and needs (Reiner,1987:51).

Those attending the victim are not the only group concerned with the patient's health and well-being. Health care personnel bring their own personal resources to encounters with patients. Whether perceived by the victims or not, support elements include instrumental-expressive dimensions from a community of people interacting together to preserve life. *Our concern here is how quality health care buffers the impact of stressful emotions.* Only recently have researchers brought this concern to the forefront of health care. From an empirical perspective, we can observe these findings and their implication that undesirable life events significantly affect depression, contemporaneously and over time. "Community and network supports do not exert a direct impact on depression, but they do seem to provide the context within which effective Strong-Tie (confidant) Support and Instrumental-Expressive Supports are formed....Psychological resources (self-esteem and personal competence) show only slight effects on change in depression" (Lin, 1987:208-209). "Females tend to show more depressive symptoms than males, and the unmarried show more depressive symptoms than do married....Marital disruption (separation, divorce, or death of a spouse) has a substantial effect on depressive symptoms. Marital disruption not only constitutes an adverse life event, but it also causes the disintegration of one's previous network of intimate and confiding ties. The effect is all the more severe for women because their intimate and confiding ties are often either restricted to their spouses or persons associated with their spouses. This double jeopardy results in longer and more sever depressive symptoms for women....History of illness (symptoms and diagnoses) shows an effect on depressive symptoms independent of undesirable life events and social support" (Lin,1986:335).

Neither health providers nor recipients should neglect the full range of personal resources. Advocates of wellness theory know how life styles can affect health and the spread of disease. Patients reap the greatest benefits from health care providers who are "an effective role model for wellness" and involve patients "in the assessment, implementation, and evaluation of wellness goals" (Clark,1986:12). Interaction facilitates learning the wholeness of health; it improves methods of care and increases responsibility for self care. Patients learn to manage life experiences, improve communication skills, and utilize social support systems.

Applied intervention does not eliminate all risks, but it gives courage through self-sufficiency. People need that to attend to harmful factors such as smoking, being overweight, high blood pressure, high cholesterol, and diabetes. Health conscious people change their life styles, decrease known risks, and reduce cardio-vascular deaths. They work with medical specialists to monitor their condition and take the proper measures as needed.

Cadavers are not resurrected by comforting words; apt phrases do not substitute for life-forces, but to activate such forces takes all the resources of personal encounters. Empathetic professionals not only listen to patients, they also motivate them (Batson and Coke, 1983:430-431). The most consistent factor in patient compliance and satisfaction is the relationship between provider and recipient. These skills are learned, yet "these skills can fade or diminish over time" (Harrigan and Rosenthal, 1987:38). Preclinical skills need updating as professionals later confront patients face-to-face. "Communication is essential in establishing rapport and is required in interviewing, the physical examination, prescribing medications, therapy, patient education, counseling and psychotherapy" (Harrigan and Rosenthal, 1987:38). Since each new patient presents a unique new challenge, professionals never finish fine-tuning their interpersonal skills, or at least they should not.

Emotional Crisis

While still in medical school in 1936, Selye noticed that sick patients had common symptoms: weight loss, physical weakness, droopy appearance, and loss of appetite. He referred to them as the "sick syndrome." In medical diagnosis, or anticipation of it, sick patients experience a host of emotions: anxiety, depression, and elation. Sickness, diagnosis, and emotions are spontaneously expressed by words or facial contortions, but to understand this dimension it meant that Selye first had to recognize these emotions and later communicate with patients appropriately. The art of communication in health care either contributes to the recovery or, through a lack of communication, complicates the situation. As Norman Cousins states, there is "a vast and growing literature on the role of the emotions and stress in opening the human body to breakdown and disease." Encounters between patients and professionals either work to alleviate illness or intensify pain.

Not all aspects of health care are physical. Fifty percent of visits for primary care are probably for psychosocial reasons, giving added importance to the physician's development of "interpersonal behavior toward patients, sensitivity to patients' emotional needs, and a pleasing bedside manner" (DiMatteo, Prince, and Hays, 1987:77). In the 19th century, physicians exhibited such skills in the face of limited medical technology. Now, however, those skills are often neglected because of medical technology. According to Eisenberg, patients still want "time, sympathetic attention, and concern for themselves as people." Health care is charged with the emotions of individuals. Emotional crises require people who care about people. Personal encounters produce emotional reactions: mild and intense, verbal and nonverbal, rational and instinctive, spontaneous and learned. Personal encounters express the inner self, that person hidden deep within the clothed.

Veninga (1985:118-129) records several ways that people destroy and build up one another. The unprepared suffer greater damage than the prepared, but the preparation must be of a certain kind. Those prepared for success in life may not necessarily be prepared for failure or sickness, tragedy or disappointment. After serious accidents, emotions may destroy family members who act as if nothing happened. Exposed wounds heal faster than hidden ones. Unresponsive individuals find tragedies extremely disturbing. Learning to share hurts can heal; silence kills.

Just as people can ignore emotions, they may also magnify them. Veninga found that exaggerators confuse threats with the real thing. Like the boy who cried "wolf, wolf," they experience the trauma of crisis emotions all the time. Those individuals that

Veninga calls Game Players either ignore or blame one another. All of these behaviors tend to destroy life and health. People can also build up one another. "Healthy families pull together, assess the damage, and plan for their future. Healthy families recognize that each member has something to contribute in overcoming a disappointment"(Veninga, 1985:131).

Figure 7-1 summarizes the stages of emotions after a disruption, a time when personal encounters mean the most. Three terms are used in this figure: certainty, accuracy, and necessity. These labels categorize emotive patterns before and after an illness. As a category, "certainty" refers to that anticipatory, emotional state of dread, fear, and anxiety by which people anticipate illnesses or injury.

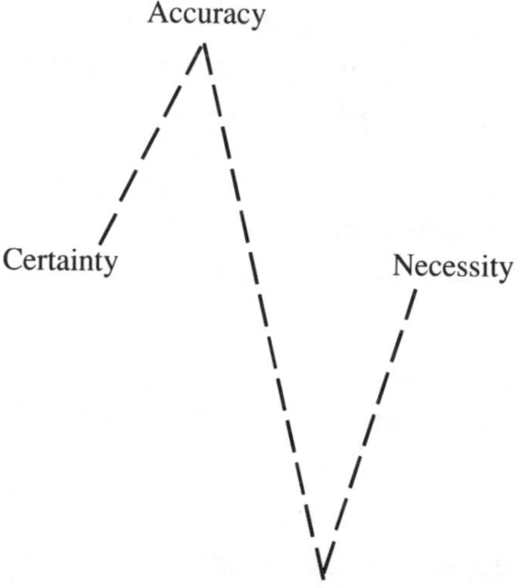

Figure 7-1. Emotional Stability Through Quality Health Care

Unfortunately, intruders disrupt health and wholeness; that's a certainty of life. To the right of certainty are dashes representing emotions, which go up and then down. This pattern symbolizes what happens to a person after the intruders of illness inevitably enter one's life. The upward motion of expanding emotions follows any tragedy. "Accuracy" refers to the ability of health providers to predict accurately these emotions that follow disruption. Synonyms include panic, shock, confusion, nothingness, numbness, and rage (see Chapter 4).

Figure 7-1 demonstrates the fluctuating emotions before recovery. Because of the disequilibrium of emotions, patients need professional intervention. "Necessity" refers to the providers who intervene with support and hope, necessities for recovery. The first recommendation of Puryear is to establish rapport with the patient. This is followed by assessing the problem, determining the patient's resources and strength, formulating a plan, and mobilizing the client (1979:51). Above all, the provider instills hope by promoting a positive self image and self reliance (1979:20-21). This means that health providers give support and also allow for independence. Time for bereavement and grief completes the healing cycle with the realization that sometimes the pain of emotion lasts longer than physical pain.

A Supportive Climate

Emotional health correlates with a positive, supportive climate. Healthy people prefer a healthy climate; unhealthy climates are deadly. Public health (death rates) varies with the social environment where people live. Those with higher satisfaction in marriage, friendships, and associations live longer (Anastas,1986:122). By contrast, isolated individuals such as the elderly, divorced, or widowed have a greater incidence of heart disease (1986:123). Not only do personal encounters contribute to health, so do the social climates where health care is practiced.

With the rise of programs such as health maintenance organizations (HMOs) and prepaid provider arrangements (PPAs), our society is debating the quality of health care. Many physicians and corporate managers wonder whether HMO facilities provide quality care, especially when profits and turnover are such dominant themes. The once accepted standard, expressed by the Hippocratic

Creed, appears to be giving way to competitive prices. Because of spiraling medical costs, corporate insurance executives are pushing more and more for cost-effective health care. "Last year in the US, there were 480 HMOs with 21 million members, compared with 178 HMOs with 5.7 million members in 1975" (Greer,1986:52). Whether arguing for the preventive services of routine child-care or for quality over cost, no one doubts that the industry is rapidly becoming a big business with money taking the front seat.

Most patients prefer supportive personal encounters with medical staff. However, over the past 50 years, the climate for this type of encounter has declined for several reasons: the spiraling costs of health care, a greater dependence on medical technology, the emergence of health care programs and group practice, the "business" of health care where specialists do routine tasks. Fortunately, Gibb (l961) has provided a framework for understanding and creating a supportive climate appropriate for quality health care. Gibb elaborates the characteristics of both defensive and supportive health care climates using eight years of research in small group dynamics (Table 7-1).

Table. 7-1 Characteristics of Supportive and Defensive Groups

Defensive Climate	**Supportive Climate**
1. Evaluation	1. Description
2. Control	2. Problem Orientation
3. Strategy	3. Spontaneity
4. Neutrality	4. Empathy
5. Superiority	5. Equality
6. Certainty	6. Provisionalism

Patients easily recognize a lack of quality. When professionals emphasize only facts about physical conditions and ignore personal feelings, patients can feel slighted (evaluation/description). Translated professional jargon is easier to understand; informed recipients engaged in problem-oriented exchanges will be less defensive about their lack of control (control/problem orientation). Strict adherence to rules and policies also creates a defensive climate. The third characteristic deals with the perception of openness and honesty in exchanges. These characteristics lead to more spontaneity from the patient who willingly cooperates. When these are lacking, patients become defensive.

The fourth characteristic suggests that those who empathize find patients more cooperative. Neutrality, or a seeming lack of concern, invalidates the patient's feelings. The fifth issue of superiority versus equality may be especially difficult in certain rigid hierarchy systems of the medical profession. It is difficult to treat people (staff or clients) as equals in a bureaucracy which operates exclusively on a hierarchical model. If superiors are superior in attitude, the climate will reflect those qualities as well. Finally, a defensive climate emerges whenever certainty dominates over provisionalism; this suggests that people feel better with tentative, even participative, decision-making in consideration of all the facts.

What characterizes these climates does not necessarily explain them or demonstrate their relevance to the sick, but Jourard (1971) cogently explains the dynamics from which a positive or negative encounter emerges. That dynamic depends upon the level of trust; people disclose their truest and deepest feelings only with those they perceive to be trustworthy, not with those who lack integrity. If Entralgo (1979:130-131) correctly assesses the emotional responses of patients, then those who create a positive climate might counteract these seven basic emotions of sick patients: fear of illness, rebellion against sickness, resigned surrender, active acceptance of medication, indifference to severity, needing professional help, and childishness.

The Issue of Professional Empathy

By attending a vocational program and serving an apprenticeship, the auto mechanic becomes quite proficient in making the correct diagnosis and in selecting the best treatment for your broken car. That's what they're trained to do. And so it is with the health care profession; but there is a difference between people and automobiles. The health care professionals learn much about the human body and how it works or doesn't work. Often the emotional dimensions of illness are not considered relevant or important to other more important clinical issues: "How long have you had fever?" "Where exactly is the pain?" "Did the medicine help the patient sleep or not?" These questions take precedence over how the patient feels emotionally, whether he or she accepts the illness well, what treatment preference the patient has, or why this treatment over that treatment.

Is the auto mechanic's professional detachment and objective rationality all that most patients want or even expect from health providers? Isn't that enough for most patients? After all, it can be argued that the effectiveness of a professional health care worker ultimately depends upon his or her competency as a specialist, not whether he or she is personally sympathetic. Who wouldn't rather have a competent physician as a surgeon over someone who, though sympathetic, has questionable credentials. The argument over quality of interpersonal encounters may ultimately depend upon what our definition of professionalism is.

But while definitions about professionalism may vary, few deny that the individual's emotional needs are greatest during times of illness. Sometimes just the shock of surgery or an accident can trip the emotional burglar alarm, and that alone can cause an iatrogenic illness. One study found that the rate of iatrogenic illness in one hospital was greater than the incidence of heart attacks in the general population. *The New England Journal of Medicine* published one study in which thirty-six percent of those hospitalized suffered trauma resulting from therapy and treatment (Anastas,1986:8). Although one study in a Boston teaching hospital cannot be generalized to the total population, it does indicate the importance of the patient's emotional needs. Not only is there an argument from the perspective of the patient, there is also evidence "that the quality of helping based on sympathy may often be superior to helping based upon cold rationality" (Blum,1986:12). A major component of effective doctor-patient interaction seems to be the expression of empathy and the development of rapport.

But what about empathetic nurses who tend to avoid certain types of patients because such contacts induce negative stress? There have been findings which suggest this type of response, especially when the adverse situation causes too much discomfort. Eisenberg distinguishes between action (motivation or avoidance) due to personal distress and that which is more altruistically based, drawing on strong feelings such as sympathy and empathy(1986:48). He sees empathy not only as the mediator for prosocial emotions, but also as the basis for altruism in general.

If empathy is as important to quality health care as is suggested, then what are the characteristics of those providers who exhibit it? Based on empirical research, the following four processes seem to determine the quality and extent of providers' prosocial behavior: 1) their role taking ability, 2) their assessment of patients' needs, 3) their emotional response to the need, 4) and their interpersonal problem solving skills. Those providers who can see life from the viewpoint of the patient and infer feelings (emotional reactions) from the patient are more likely to exhibit prosocial behavior. Obviously, these same abilities could lead to manipulation, depending upon the values of the provider. Second, patient assement affects the quality of the help rendered (whether the recipient cannot perform the tasks or help themselves). If patients are unable to help themselves, then the provider will more likely render help, but if the patients could help themselves, the provider is less likely to help. Attributions about the patient are a determining factor. Third, how people feel about others also determines the measure of help given. It may even depend upon stereotypes, prejudices, and attitudes toward certain minorities. If a health provider can identify with and feel positive about a patient, he or she is more likely to render the highest quality service. Finally, much of the quality of service seems to depend upon the abilities of the provider, regardless of other emotional factors, and Eisenberg believes that one's ability to come up with solutions to problems means a person at least has the ability to make the right choices.

These four differences may be due to a variety of factors, including the background training of the provider. Even with these distinctions, the proper approach can be learned once the provider becomes aware of the patient's need, knows what action to take, and has confidence in his ability to act appropriately. If these assumptions are true, then health providers can learn how to attend to the emotional as well as physical needs of patients. One suggestion is to pay attention to the obstacles of emotional release. If those obstacles aren't clear, then ask some key questions: What prevents the patient from grieving or getting feelings out in the open? What topics does the patient avoid or just won't discuss? The provider should note when clients are hesitant to interact. Why is this? What does the person seem to avoid?

The Personal Exchange

It is necessary on some occasions to communicate with clients on a personal level. While that exposure and exchange of feelings at the deepest level is risky for some, others are quite comfortable. Empathy with another person is quite paradoxical: the more a provider truly feels the other person's feelings, the less important are her own feelings. When people are "getting inside another" they are, at the same time, "getting outside themselves." Deep feelings for others only come as we lose some of the feelings for ourselves. However, to lose oneself entirely in the emotions of another is not good either, so there is a proper separation of provider from recipient, and that can be found in actions. After all, it is demonstrated behavior that underlines or crosses out what we say. The providers maintain their own feeling level in this way, while at the same time they can feel for the other person.

Significant exchanges in health care require caring attitudes and actions. They can't be separated, and shouldn't be. Muldary (1983:117-118), however, advocates that the line be drawn between professionalism and overidentification with the patient's feelings. If patients are involved at the deepest personal level in communication with health professionals, then the professionals have an obligation to reciprocate in kind. Some modified suggestions from Muldary are given below:

1) The tightness of the professional mask must be loosened enough for this type of personal exchange to occur. When providers cannot shift from the professional role to the personal role, it is often because they feel uneasy doing so.

2) Time is also a factor, for no one reveals his or her true feelings to a busy professional. It may not require a great deal of time, but not much of a conversation will ensue if there is evidence of a "hurried rush." The key is whether the professional appears relaxed and willing to engage in serious conversation.

3) There must be active listening during these occasions as well. Perhaps the best adage to describe this is "hearing is not listening." We can hear noise without paying attention to the source of that sound. The same is true for patients.

4) The professional can learn to grasp the perspective of the patient more clearly; to communicate and interpret in very subtle ways. A parent learns to interpret the particular cry of an infant; the sound, pitch, and intensity communicating exactly what the problem is. The professional must develop the same sensitivity to the cries of a patient in distress.

5) Once inside, the professional can "go back and forth," so to speak. Each round trip strengthening emotional bonding and promoting understanding. These experiences create an emotional extension of oneself, a person who can share at the very deepest level. Just as the dream is said to be the heart of

the soul, so also is the specialist the extended self, at least in these moments. Thus the reciprocal relation comes full circle; from one back to another, both benefiting from these exchanges (1983:118).

Figure 7-2 shows the uniqueness of these personal exchanges. It represents the personal exchange between provider and recipient in terms of the depth of communication. A professional may communicate empathy (German word *einfulung*, "feeling into") or she may not. A patient may or may not disclose his or her true feelings. The four boxes in the figure represent the various combinations of these encounters between professional and patient. Starting with the upper left box and moving across, we can see part of the dynamics of these exchanges. For example, one type of exchange is represented when neither the professional nor the patient shows his or her feelings, an "impersonal exchange." The next box to the right indicates a "personal exchange" in that the professional takes off the mask and gives time for serious feedback; however, the patient is still unwilling to disclose his or her feelings.

Professional Empathy

	No	Yes
No Patient's Sympathy	Impersonal Exchange	Personal Exchange
Yes	Impersonal Encounter	Personal Encounter

Figure 7-2. Emotional Exchange Between Provider and Recipient.

As in the top row, so will it be in the bottom row across. In this case the patient is willing to open up, but the professional may or may not. When the professional does not take the time, does not listen, or does not remove his or her mask, the encounter is impersonal. By contrast, however, when both the patient and the professional enter into deeper channels where true feelings reside, that is when personal encounters begin. These rare moments are difficult to achieve and risky at best.

Gazda et al. (1982) suggest some precautions for health professionals attempting this type of interaction, especially in regard to stress. Such personal encounters are demanding and draining emotionally; the helpers often need help themselves. Professionals who achieve this type of client relation experience "burn out" quicker than those who do not.

Professionals should also be alert for patients who refuse to open up or who are from a different culture. They may need to seek help or advice from another professional. Finally, even though these encounters are rarely achieved, they can become a source of satisfaction because such encounters confirm the purpose of the professional's job, a commitment to help others return to health and wholeness once again.

Emotional Transfer and Release

Before a patient goes to a clinic for treatment, several decisions must be made: who to see, where to go, what to do, how to pay, when to start, and why the problem. There is a transfer of emotions between recipient and provider which develops from both the decisions and exchanges between the two. The recipient has pain, mourns, hurts, and experiences a deep need like that of hunger, which explains why they seek help. Based on these needs, the provider sees the patient, listens to what is said, touches the feelings of hurt, and shares the needs of the patient. The basic exchange begins on the physical level because of a biological dysfunction, but the illness also has psychosocial qualities. What begins with sense perceptions evolves into social definitions. Sense perception is important because that is where the patient comes from and where the dialogue begins. It is determined by feelings expressed by the patient: discomfort, pain, feelings of uneasiness. These are subjective, social, and cultural in character, but they affect perceptions, interpretations, and explanations.

The provider begins and sometimes ends with the social aspects of an illness. This suggests that both content (medical advice) and style (manner delivered) of interaction become important factors in determining the final outcome. Of course, during these discussions, those in attendance should speak slowly and clearly, giving reassurance whenever possible. If there is negative or destructive behavior, then limit that, but don't argue. Minimize loud noises or sudden interruptions. Emotional support through personal encounters frequently improves dispositions, if for nothing more than acceptance of reality. Adjustment is then possible, one with less anxiety over the changes. Emotional synergy may or may not be outwardly visible; therefore it should not be the basis for action or interaction.

Personal, intimate encounters never teach people about the intricate details of microbiology or physiology. Those facts are learned through specialized curricula at the undergraduate and graduate levels. While such training is essential to health care, it does not give much attention to the emotional side of health care. That's unfortunate, because personal encounters give us an understanding of humanness that can't be found anywhere else.

It is difficult to understand how the emotions of others can mean so much if we have never lost something or someone very meaningful to us. From these personal, emotional experiences can come a healthy respect for others. In extreme cases, however, failure to control a strong emotional outburst can still occur, but that comes with the job. As Maspach expressed it, "More experienced health care people are surprisingly silent on this topic and do not share their own experience with younger colleagues, which suggests that the prevailing philosophy is one of paying your dues"(1979:115). Even so, these emotional experiences serve as vital links between the provider and the recipient in health care services.

Emotional release and transfer come best as the provider renders the action suggested above, but research has confirmed that non-verbal cues help considerably. Janis (1983:90-91) reviewed the literature to find which nonverbal cues are most highly correlated with positive emotional transfer and release of the client:

1) Bodily face the person when talking with them.
2) Lean toward them slightly in conversations.
3) Maintain eye contact during interaction.
4) Smile, bite lips slightly, and open mouth.
5) Nod your head up and down as they speak.
6) Sit straight and keep hands down on lap.
7) Listen often but speak clearly when appropriate.

Janis summarizes the importance of personal encounters this way: 1) Give realistic information to patients. If they deny the reality of the situation, then work with them gently to challenge their "blanket immunity reassurances" (1983:191); 2) After you know the patient and their strengths, then it is appropriate to recognize those strengths both individually and socially. What have they got going for them? These strokes counteract negative emotional feelings. 3) Encourage them to work out their own problems with the resources they have. You, as the provider of health care, must counter the tendency toward passivity and inactivity. This may require the learning of new coping skills not previously recognized or realized. The role of the professional is crucial to utilizing the emotional intervention necessary to overcome the stress of illness or loss.

Health Professionals as Mentors

Too much giving, without the regeneration of expended emotions, can itself be stressful. That's why the concept of mentors is important. A mentor is a senior professional who voluntarily and spontaneously assumes a personal, yet mutually beneficial relationship with a junior professional. It is an emotional relationship characterized by strong loyalty. Since the frequent interaction with one another tends to be rather exclusive, management's acceptance of this quality of mentoring is an important aspect of its development. Other factors can hinder development of mentor relationships. If a work environment emphasizes production, then mentors must contribute to that purpose or run contrary to the organization climate. As health care in general, and hospital services in particular, becomes more profit than people centered, mentor roles, along with quality health care may disappear in the future.

There are four diverse types of mentor relationships. They can be described as coach, developer, leader, and sponsor; each fulfills an important function for junior professionals. The coach imparts knowledge and skills to the understudy. The developer inspires strong sentiments and feelings about professionalism and its responsibilities. The leader instills character qualities; if he is a leader in the true sense of the word. Finally, the sponsor promotes the junior mentor and shows her not only where the opportunities are, but how to access the network.

Mentoring benefits health care workers in many ways, not the least of which is the protection from stressors. It is a fact that prolonged patient care, common to the health care fields, increases the likelihood of burnout. Mentor relationships protect not only the patient during times of illness, but also the providers in times of their own personal stress. For if patients experience high levels of emotional stress, surely those providing health care will also be affected. Maslanch (1979:114-119) has made this very point in a study on burnout syndrome and patient care. Given the likelihood of such an experience, he found various ways in which health care professionals cope with the tendency towards burnout: learning more about emotional elements, understanding distressing experiences, gaining support from associates, using humor as a release, separating work and play, and maintaining good physical health. All of these strategies have been valuable for other health professionals.

At the 1986 American Management Association Conference in

San Francisco, William Sackett described some of the difficulties that could develop with mentoring: jealousy from professionals, resentment among peers, and tensions in personal relationships. There is always the possibility that all the negative aspects of the senior professional might be transferred to the junior member. There can also be an unprofitable investment of time and energy which results in few professional or personal gains, a serious problem among professionals who value their limited time and resources. Finally, Sackett suggests that perceived intimacy and loyalty can be fake; producing dependency, especially in those cases involving strong senior professionals.

Tips in Health Service

For intervention to be effective, patients and providers should understand their roles. Currently prescribed medicine and the authority of attending medical personnel take precedence, but there will be opportunities to take alternative approaches. Implementation of those approachs depends more upon the patient than the provider. It can help to clarify role expectations by asking the patient "What do you expect from me?" or "What do you hope to achieve now?" Through role clarification, each person knows more clearly what is expected.

Obviously, listening attentively helps in knowing what to do or how to act. Listen for more than words; try to get to the meaning the words convey, but also remember some basic ideas about guiding the patient to be more creative. Influenced by W. Paul Torrance, Henderson and Bryan (1984:256-257) list some valuable tips for those charged with assisting another. They have direct application for health care professionals and are presented here in a modified form.

1) "Wanting to know." Providers must help patients to determine what they want to know. Find out where their curiosity lies.

2) "Digging deeper." Providers must not give pat answers in difficult situations. Let patients dig deeper for themselves rather than give superficial answers.

3) "Looking twice and listening for smells." Providers must realize the rights of the patient to look twice and listen for smells. A patient's struggling for a sense of well-being can be healthy.

4) "Listening for the cat." Providers must learn how to communicate nonverbally. Patients communicate with more than just words.

5) "Crossing out mistakes." Providers should allow their patients to explore new strategies. Don't discourage patients when they want to risk new approaches, allow them to fail.

6) "Getting into and out of deep water." Providers should allow patients to select from alternative intervention strategies. Allow them to venture out on their own.

7) "Having a ball." Providers should allow their patients time for relaxation.

8) "Cutting a hole to see through." Providers should give positive feedback to patients whenever possible.

9) "Building sand castles." Providers should encourage their patients to dream.

10) "Singing in your own key." Providers should accept their patients even when they deviate from others.

11) "Plugging in the sun." Providers should learn about new intervention strategies or technologies which might help their patients recover in the most rapid manner.

12) "Shaking hands with the future." Providers must realize their transient role and be prepared to accept others who also need their services.

So far we have discussed the changes in terminology (patient's needs), and then the changes in the provider's role of prescribing some positive action. Now let's give attention to the partnership between provider and patients in light of this discussion. A partnership means just that—a joint effort by more than one person. The implications for this type of arrangement in any emotive therapy have been recognized by Hoff (1984:113-115). She listed the basic management strategy for working in partnership with a person or family in crisis:

1) Develop with the person in crisis. It is a collaborative effort. Don't do for others what they can do for themselves.

2) Be problem oriented. Take the immediate concrete problems first, then go to the more complex matters. In other words, set priorities, do the most important things first.

3) Be appropriate to functional levels and dependency needs. Assess how the person feels, copes, and acts; then react accordingly. Above all, don't force dependency upon anyone.

4) Be consistent with people's culture and life style. People vary as much by class, religion, beliefs, values, and language as they do in how they respond to the critical events of life, death, accidents, injury, and illness.

5) Include significant other(s) and the social network. Always involve those most directly connected to the patient. "Since crises occur when there is a serious disruption in normal social transactions, or in the way one perceives oneself in the social milieu, planning must attend to these important social factors" (Hoff:1984:115).

Sometimes an agreement worked out between the provider and patient helps. The agreement is, of course, voluntary and other factors should be considered:

1) What does the client expect from the counselor?
2) What does the counselor expect from the client?
3) How do the two parties achieve their expected goals?

4) How do they implement target dates for achieving these goals (Hoff:1984:117)?

The purpose of this chapter is to increase human understanding in stressful situations. We must be aware of the unintended and un-recognized reactions between provider and recipient. There is a mediating process—the degree of empathy with the patient. In today's equation of sociomedical intervention, attention is directed toward the science of medicine and away from the art, but it was that art which served us well in the past. Providers can combine that art with modern technology to have a better picture of what the patient's needs are.

Chapter 8

Intervention Strategies During Recovery

After a near miss, the nervous pilot once again deliberately intervenes. Until this need for recovery of attention, the pilot flew the plane with mind and emotions on automatic. Recognizing the outside world without full attention is how most of us drive. Once things become familiar, once they are categorized for reaction, then our attention is diverted to other things. Driving that way is less fatiguing because it doesn't require full attention, but like the pilot, we can run into problems. For the pilot not to notice what does not fit is dangerous; when the unfamiliar obstacle suddenly appears in front of the plane, it demands full attention. Survival is instinctive; to give our full attention or no attention depends upon the danger in a situation (Maslow:1954:205-209).

Until the need for recovery of attention, the pilot flew with a sort of free floating attention. In the beginning of pilot training, the fear of flying distracts the student pilot's full attention away from important details. To overcome these fears of flying is not easy, especially after a close midair encounter with death, but it can be done if the pilots not only confront their fears, but correct their errors. These pilots need practical emotional intervention strategies. Emergency simulation tests are one such method used to help the pilots practice those procedures that must be performed quickly and accurately during an emergency. It is an example of an intervention technique that helps an individual learn to control his emotions, especially in an emergency.

What works for pilots can also work for patients during their recovery from serious injury or illness. Intervention strategies develop practical emotional procedures to help patients in crisis situations. One intervention alleviates patient suffering from stress; the other reduces the number who suffer from diseases. One is preventive; the other curative. To use either effectively depends upon how providers match strategies to patients. That's the challenge to health care providers: to assess not only the needs of patients, but also the appropriateness of interventions. To understand what disturbs patients we can observe the following: their inability to learn certain tasks, their indifference to satisfactory relations, their propensity to complain about physical symptoms or fears, their inconsistency in adjusting to certain situations, and their tendency to be passive or inactive. Techniques of diagnosis change with intervention strategies and concepts, both of which are covered in this chapter.

Analogical Guidelines

Health professionals follow certain steps in assessing their patients. They establish clear procedures which multidisciplinary medical teams use to coordinate interdisciplinary work. Gogler has developed an emergency categories scheme which sets priorities for treatment. Those who treat trauma victims initially give attention to the "ABCs" (airway, breathing, circulation). Unfortunately, the socioemotional side of patients is not as easy to monitor as the biophysical side. X-rays and CT scans don't work for emotions. That type of analysis depends more on the art of medicine rather than the science. What follows is one procedure which could be used to evaluate the socioemotional dynamics of patients.

There are six questions and four areas of concern in the "64 Formula" used to evaluate patients. The six questions—who, what, how, when, where, and why—fit into one of four areas: 1) focus (who and what), 2) progress (how), 3) practical matters (when and where), and 4) legal and ethical issues (why). We first consider the target of intervention; "what" is the person's greatest vulnerability? Major affected areas should be identified as targets for changing behavior or life-style, and patients should understand alternatives. Second, providers set up complete accounting systems to determine "how" as progress develops. Both patients and support members must agree about how progress is to be measured. The third area deals with practical matters such as adjustments after surgery or extended illness. The fourth area of the 64 formula includes legal and ethical issues which overlap into the "why" questions. It might mean redefining or reexamining the needs of the patient.

The 64 formula is no substitute for knowing patients. Readiness and motivation are the keys, so that encouragement of positive behavior may make a difference. Never mistake emotions that are difficult to control for motivations that are necessary for recovery. Providers can assist patients in making this distinction. Although anxiety may begin the process of recovery, motivation is what keeps the recovery going. Patients will never solve motivation problems until they substitute positive activities for negative anxieties.

Providers and recipients must work together. Providers give reassurance, attentiveness, sympathy, and inspiration which promote a positive and open partnership. They intervene and use analogies as motivation tools. Psychotherapists, for example, teach wheelchair patients how to interact with others, anticipating that need as part of their future. First sessions involve group games. These games simulate conflicts which require patients to make decisions, seek assistance, and in the process, begin to feel good about themselves. After this initial stage, the social training then moves to actual social settings. However, emotions remain problematic: "Increasing numbers of patients with depressive symptoms prompted staff of the Bad Hearing Rehabilitation Center to establish a self-help program against depressive attitudes in the form of group therapy" (Strubreither,1987:215).

Emotive Propellents

During illness or after life threatening injuries, patients need added strength. People naturally feel helpless and overcome. It is not uncommon for people to "enter an emotional state due to an interaction between certain situational factors and differing personal traits. If he or she is also the emotionally reactive type, this emotional state can be expected to be extended (both in magnitude or duration)" (Melamed,1987:224). Those individuals cope best with elevated blood pressure, for example, who know their strengths and capacities, as well as those of others. It helps if providers, family members, and friends buffer the afflicted until patients get reoriented emotionally. After a loss, patients adapt and recover before positive emotions propel them once again (See Figure 8-1).

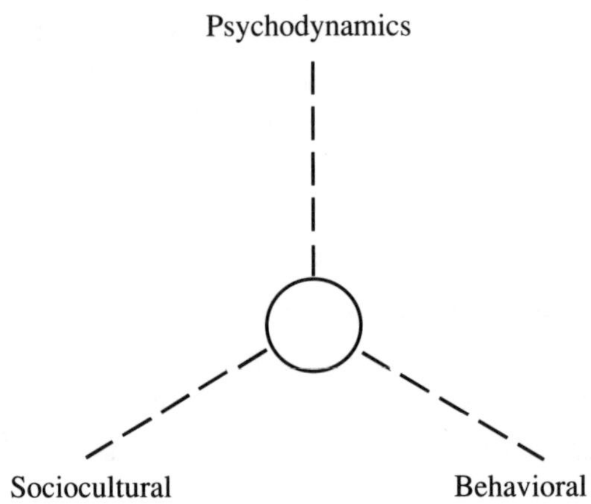

Figure 8-1. The Emotive Propeller.

The dynamics of emotional energy form the basis for psychosocial life. These energies—psychodynamics, behavioral, and sociocultural—propel traumatized patients during their recovery. If an airplane develops mechanical problems, they are fixed; the off-center propeller screw gets tightened; propeller efficiency (thrust to energy) is analyzed. After basic adjustments (physical), then mechanics routinely check for blade pitch and speed (emotions) to ensure that the plane will now fly properly. The same two forces—physical and emotional—are the energy which propels patients into recovery. The plane takes off and flies only if the engine and propeller work. With mechanical problems, however, no amount of prodding from others overcomes the laws of aerodynamics.   The age of the patient determines much. Children have more to lose than 90-year-olds; mothers with young worry more than singles without children. "Women are more concerned about the effect of their disability on their personal relationships and responsibilities" (Salby and Glicksman,1985:203). Social factors vary, but general principles remain constant; each emotive blade in Figure 8-1 has its own intervention strategies to insure the proper functioning of other parts. Providers can encourage patients to manage their problems, to understand the basic principles of psychodynamics, and to acquire social competency which buffers them from further complications.

Psychodynamics

Patients desire independent living and control of their environment. Loss of control affects people in different ways, but everyone wonders how much has been lost. "What can't be done now that could have been done before?" Each time this question is asked, an outburst of emotions usually follows. Figure 8-1 describes how providers can use information with their patients. Psychodynamics refers to uncontrollable physiological changes that take place during and after a medical problem. These changes follow predictable cycles of alarm, resistance, and exhaustion, as shown by the general adaption syndrome (Selye, 1976). Psychodynamics deals with the emotions of anxiety, depression, and autonomic arousal commonly associated with major change events.

Providers can explain how traumatic experiences produce predictable emotional responses. These responses develop as function decreases and dependency increases. No one likes being dependent upon others, but during the chaos of crises, patients require direct intervention. They may neither think clearly nor act normally. By being sensitive to patients, the health care team assists immediately following crises. As the patient regains independence, he or she returns to normality, but some patients may require additional counseling. The role of psychodynamics is one of three parts of the emotive propeller; the behavioral and sociocultural factors of recovery make up the other two.

Behavioral

Much has been written about the effect of life styles on individual health. By conservative estimates, 10 million Americans have a drinking problem; 40 million are overeaters; and approximately 55 million smoke. Perhaps the best known studies relating life style to health deal with the Type A personality: individuals who are extremely impatient, restless, competitive, explosive, tense, responsible, active, and anxious about time pressures. This type of personality has been linked to risk for heart disease. More directly related to patient care is the fact that half of the patients who make appointments in this country do not keep them. Failure to intervene with life style changes can disastrously affect successful recovery. This is also true for the sociocultural category.

Sociocultural

To intervene with significant others is wise because of the importance of their support. Exactly how they provide support depends upon how much patients are affected physically. Providers can ask questions to determine the appropriate networks: Can they go to school, work, or handle normal responsibilities? How have relationships been affected? Is there someone or a group to which the patient can turn if needed? Or is the former support system gone, altered, or inappropriate? The family and other support systems can either buffer the person or contribute to further emotional problems, depending upon the circumstances. Job, marriage, work overload, status inconsistency—all of these affect relationships and well-being.

There are also cultural dimensions. Health care workers understand patients by these social factors: ethnic groups, religion, race, and values of reference groups. Since these indicate how people might respond to death, divorce, illness, pregnancy/abortion, or accidents; social indicators should be used in intervention strategies. Care is significantly related to these communal aspects, especially when dealing with any type of loss. When someone has compounding problems—illness, accidents, death, loss—that person needs all the support that is available. Loss of health, job, home, or a loved one, in conjunction with additional health problems, makes the selection of intervention strategies all the more important.

Adaptations begin with the family. In life-threatening illnesses, Slaby and Glicksman have found that "the entire family is involved in the treatment process" (1985:177). Whenever the patient loses control or the ability to respond to treatment, then the whole family is severely affected. Exactly how patients respond varies: some strike out in anger; others see their own frailties and weaknesses.

Many would agree with the suggestion that health care intervention be extended beyond the individual level where contact is usually made. Rueveni et al. (1982) argued for a more encompassing involvement of health care with others (family, friends, neighbors, personal support groups). This would take some of the burden away from individuals and make the problem of providing health care more consistent with its true characteristics.

Many crises are community-related, described by patterns of social disintegration. That disintegration may be temporary or become chronic, depending upon the problem, but crisis inevitably involves others. Some social factors which increase stress and anxiety include alcoholism, suicides, mental breakdowns, and dysfunctional families. Non-traditional intervention strategies are needed, if for no other reason than that the magnitude of the problem is too great for the traditional health professionals. If two out of every ten Americans are in serious need of some type of mental health service, then interventions will have to be redirected toward those support groups already in place.

Rational Approach

Whether the individual's problems are serious or not, there is a logical approach to intervention during recovery. Figure 8-2 lists the key rational elements in the "Program Data" acrostic.

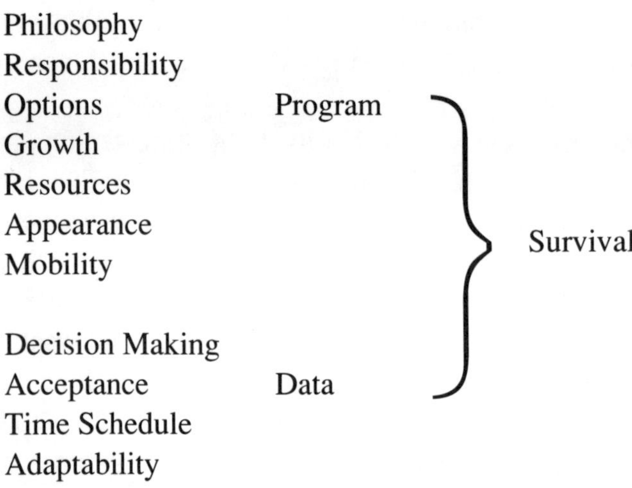

Figure 8-2. Program Data for Survival

Eisenson (1984:258) lists some of the adjustment needs of patients and their families: changes in role relationship between members and their corollary altered life style; practical problems related to financial problems, neglect of jobs, health matters; emotional adjustments which deal with irritability, anger, guilt, oversolicitousness, and rejection. His research suggests that both rational and emotional adjustments form the basis for any intervention.

Before focusing on a particular patient need, providers should make clear their *philosophy* of patient care—to help them help themselves, to encourage them to be self sufficient, to make clear all the relevant health care facts. Extending from that philosophy, providers develop an intervention strategy: determining *responsibility*, considering the *options*, assessing the personal *growth*, locating available *resources*, evaluating physical *appearance*, and selecting a type of *mobility*. However, this program requires additional data: making *decisions*, *acceptance* of a program, a *time schedule* of bench marks, and *adaptability* to new and previously unexpected challenges. Only by combining both of these—program and data—do providers match the best intervention to their patients.

Once "program data" is understood by the patient, then both the provider and the recipient can proceed to establish goals and appropriate behavior. Intervention can then begin on a positive note. Knowing where and how to start is important, for patients ultimately determine their own success, but only if they are committed to the program and intend to follow it. Once targets are established, then collaborators should agree on some deadlines from which to chart progress. These targeted changes should promote health, improve adjustments in the immediate social setting, improve skills, and increase development. However evident the intentions, motivation to act remains the key to successful completion. Of course positive reinforcement from those providing health care helps. So do self-recording activities where the recipient records progress in a diary.

Lazarus states that program data should increase the patient's coping abilities, and that may depend upon the problem solving stage, a stage much like the rational one just discussed. He lists the following areas to be dealt with in the problem solving stage: 1) coping with reality and the way things really are; 2) learning to state your problems and ask for help; 3) attacking the problem in smaller, more controllable portions; 4) trusting others for their advice; 5) being confident about the outcome. During severe illnesses and emergencies, however, the rational approach initially tends to break down, and a subjective response emerges (Slaikeu,1984:18).

Lessons from Emergencies

In natural or human-made disasters, professionals observe a variety of community responses to such conditions as grief and mourning, emergencies, suicide, illnesses, terminal illnesses, wars, death, and dying. Field studies of these experiences, unlike laboratory research, contribute to "the facilitation of an important human concern: "coping with stress" (Kobasa, 1982:26). These studies also isolate the subjective components of stress: how people handle positive and negative feelings; and how communities cope with stress at several levels and control it (Slaikeu, 1984:18). Relief workers know that people openly express strong emotional feelings during tragedies. They have seen people both openly cry out in pain and warmly show gratitude to others. It is not uncommon for victims to feel "great surges of love for family, friends, acquaintances, and even strangers" (Kliman, et al., 1982:258). Should stress already exist before these events, these feelings are compounded.

People under extreme stress have limits as to what they can handle. When those limits are exceeded, victims may deny the problem or be unable emotionally to assess it. Psychic numbing can be an indication of emotional overloading. Whether there is numbing or denial, many signs show the disaster's impact: irritation, anxiety, tensions, anger. Those in disasters, reflecting illness behavior, often show major signs of depression: 1) no appetite, loss of weight; 2) insomnia; 3) psychomotor agitation; 4) social withdrawal; 5) lack of energy; 6) feelings of worthlessness; 7) inattentiveness, poor concentration; and 8) recurrent thoughts of death. In the DSM-III scale, victims or patients characterized by any four of these meet the criteria of major depression (Feuerstein, Labbe, Kuczmierczyk, 1987:308). Compounded emotions are even more difficult to overcome.

Severe losses scar victims emotionally and leave them in a state of rage because of the "loss of self-worth," especially if the event is human-made (Kliman, et al., 1982:259). Even though routine surgery may not be as catastrophic as disasters, it too disrupts patterns and produces uncommon emotions. For this reason, Purtilo recommends that health professionals get below the cliche level in conversations with patients and discover appropriate interventions. Providers do that by encouraging the patient to talk about themselves. They can use questions such as the following to open up communication:

1) What wounds or hurts do you resent having suffered?
2) What gifts were you given for which you were most grateful?
3) Who are your important heroes and models?
4) What were the crucial decisions for which you were responsible?

These questions prompt people to release their frustrations and to redirect their emotions. However, those who have been victimized and brutalized experience "psychopathology, regardless of their prior level of functioning" (Purtilo, 1982:271). The stress of disaster pains those afflicted; they experience painful adaptation. Emotions of pain—depression, anxiety—regulate the social bonds in mammals, primates, and humans. After disasters, victims readily adapt to the dependency state of helplessness. They increase interaction and social communication. This effort compensates for fluctuating emotions which are dependent upon high self-esteem and good self-image.

Recent research has given us a number of insights regarding emotional encounters. Emotions fluctuate as people relive the stressful events. Dependence brings relief through interaction with others, and that interaction comes in many forms. Emotional recovery comes as people share—anger, guilt, anxiety, frustration, fear, depression. Sharing diffuses excessive feelings that make adjustment more difficult (Klerman and Weissman, 1985:55-76). Studies of relaxation training have shown a 28 percent reduction in reported pain. Relaxation brings relief by controlling excessive reactions. It helps for people to share their emotional feelings with sympathetic others; the pain of emotions will come out, and people should not remain silent during crises (Feuerstein, Labbe, Kuczmierczyk, 1987:308). All of these insights can help to improve quality of health care.

While originally designed to analyze chronic pain, the following list of questions may also be useful in cases of emotional pain:

1) Describe your pain experiences throughout a typical day.
2) Which activities or events bring on or increase your pain?
3) List the activities or techniques which decrease your experience of pain.
4) What physical, social, and work activities have been altered because of your pain problem?
5) Which of these would you like to resume?
6) If I were in the room and your were in pain, how would I know?
7) What would you do or say?
8) How does your spouse react when you're in pain?
9) What do you do in response to his or her pain?

The very process of thinking about and answering these questions helps the patient in "learning pain reduction and stress reduction techniques that can substitute for conventional strategies (Feuerstein, Labbe, Kuczmierczyk, 1987:466-467).

Besides the opportunity for sharing feelings, there is another important factor related to recovery. What people believe about the future relates to their ability to dream about something beyond the tragedies. Religious beliefs are another factor determining how people handle their crises. These beliefs continue throughout recovery as people make practical decisions about interventions. The social composition of the support group is still another factor in recovery; homogeneous groups show less conflict,especially in the matter of beliefs and values. The natural group also provides greater support because these people are already in the social network. Natural group gatherings work best because people empathize with others and their feelings. Finally, the interactive group works best. On the whole, there must be an active rather than passive approach to tragic events, for only then are people able to counter feelings of isolation, abandonment and guilt, and decrease feelings of helplessness and low self-esteem.

People increase interaction and social communication as they respond to emotional trauma, solicit expressions, and direct new feelings in a positive way. The intensity of that interaction depends upon basic needs: 1) to maintain a sense of trust, 2) to avoid diffuse anxiety and 3) to sustain self-concept. These three needs are met by a sense of group inclusion, ontological security, and symbolic/material gratifications. As people present themselves to others and negotiate with others they show a readiness to comply. Their "sense of facticity will be more strongly influenced by efforts to avoid the anxiety associated with a failure to sustain self and create a sense that things are as they are" (Turner,1987:25). Security about how things are, trust or dependence on others, and group inclusion are significantly related to the sincerity and genuineness of how one is presented to others. Any disruption in life demands that people redefine their social and physical worlds, along with their own sense of identity. That is why social interventions are important, because there is a tendency to explain motivation only in cognitive processes, not as interpersonal motivation (Turner, 1987:15).

Alternative Approaches for Coping

Gordon (1982:22) found that many patients in the psychiatric emergency ward could be treated at home. Here their problems could be seen in the social context where they actually occurred. With help from a team of health professionals made up of nurses, paraprofessionals, and psychologists, he provided service at the point of origin. From those experiences, Gordon has identified some characteristics of alternative interventions that he feels are important:

1) Respond to people's problems as experienced. Evaluate the social setting where the problem originates.
2) Provide services at the point of crisis; don't wait until going to the hospital.
3) See problems as opportunities in which change and development are occurring, "even psychotic episodes are regarded as potentially transformative." The role of drugs is down-played.
4) Always see anyone coming for help as part of a network or clan.
5) From the beginning, start sharing responsibility within the patient's support group.
6) Be open to other mental health techniques and alternative approaches, especially community-based approaches.
7) Make the recipient take responsibility for his or her own problem. Listen to suggestions about how to help.

Gordon extends traditional interventions with these recommendations. These recommendations involve people with similar problems who give time to others. These programs are community-based, involving some paraprofessionals, but many more lay people. Their service record is "equal or superior to that offered by traditional mental health services" (Gordon,1982:26).

Alternative approaches are designed to assist adults and children in different ways. Providers working with adults first evaluate the environment of those needing help. By lending a hand, providers can perhaps be agents of change. One strategy is to encourage recipients to set limited goals in the early stages. This fosters hope through expectations, a factor designed to counter hopelessness. Both provider and recipient engage supporters whenever possible. All of these people work together to plan for the future, while not neglecting the past. They promote worthiness and self-esteem whenever possible, encourage independence and self-reliance, and listen attentively (Hafen, Peterson, and Frandsen, 1982:11-13).

While these suggestions work for adults, they may not work for children. When dealing with children, providers are more flexible and indirect in their approach. While honest with their own emotions, providers realize that the emotions of children are temporary in nature. Providers accept the extreme reactions of children for what they are. That means allowing the child much physical rest; sessions are kept short, yet long enough to be truthful about the topics. Adults who already know the children are more likely to protect them from harsh realities, while at the same time provide an atmosphere of care and support (Hafen, et al.1982:13-14).

Recent studies have highlighted the pressing need for coping strategies among the Vietnam ara veterans. Overwhelmed by their experiences in Vietnam, these veterans struggle with their combat experience and post-service trauma. In a study on mortality, researchers found that Vietnam veterans reached 17 percent higher levels of mortality than veterans of others wars (CDC,1987). Clinicians wondered what factors intensify or buffer postraumatic stress. *Selecting ten from a sample 100 veterans, two psychiatrists isolated the counteractive qualities which buffered veterans from excessive trauma.* First, intensive clinical evaluations were performed. Then, they identified those veterans with emotionally protective qualities. The researchers described five protective qualities that they observed: 1) the ability to function calmly under pressure; 2) belief in understanding and judgment; 3) acceptance of fear in self and others; 4) lack of excessive violence; and 5) the absence of guilt. The authors conclude from these ten case studies that future studies on stressful conditions should examine "perceptual and adaptive factors, rather than simply objective aspects of the combat experience...that it is not so much what the individual experienced in Vietnam, but how those events and situations were perceived, integrated, and acted on that bears the primary relationship to the postcombat response" (Hendin and Haas, 1984).

The Social Basis of Empowerment

Garfield (1979) contends that sympathetic and supportive associations induce health because these relationships provide people with an incentive to live. That disposition correlates with increased chances of survival. Quoting a past president of the American Cancer Society, Dr. Eugene P. Pendergrass believes "there is solid evidence that the course of disease in general is effected by emotional distress....Thus, we, as doctors, may begin to emphasize treatment of the patient as a whole, as well as the disease from which the patient is suffering" (1979:5).

Support for this idea was found in a study of long-term physical illnesses in children. The researcher examined the psychosocial adaptations that occur simultaneously with such illnesses. The findings suggest that success in managing the child's condition really depended upon two significant groups:

1) The continuous "personalized" support and counseling by the physician, who should be alert to all the incompatible feelings with which both the patient and his parents are coping.

2) The parents' acceptance of the disease with its uncertain course and impact on the family, implying that they had gradually mastered their conflicting emotions, aroused by their child's ailment (Mattsson, 1979:260).

The issue of empowerment for the disabled or chronically ill has become an increasingly important issue (Henderson and Bryan, 1984:vii). Some thirty million people suffer from disabilities or chronic illnesses of one type or another. How can we as a country promote the work ethic while at the same time failing to design more jobs for those that are chronically disabled, but who want to work? Henderson and Bryson believe that much of our thinking about these individuals is culturally and socially biased. Their suggestions for redesign of our social system include the following observations:

1) People with disabilities are showing themselves as having power.
2) People with disabilities are asking for more positions of authority in agencies established to assist them.
3) People with disabilities want more positive images of themselves in the electronic media.
4) People with disabilities are developing a marketing identity.

Too often these people, along with others having emotional problems, experience problems in adjustment. This occurs in one of five ways: 1) physical or emotional stigma; 2) individual abilities; 3) disabilities; 4) social barriers; and 5) life activities. As a result of these barriers, the general public does not understand their condition. For example, people don't feel comfortable with these people; they don't know how to treat them; and these individuals often become social outcasts as a result (Henderson and Bryan, 1984:84-93).

After loss, people go through a transitional state during which they build their fences. A fence serves a dual purpose: it keeps out insolent neighbors, but keeps in courteous ones. Each type of neighbor has an effect on the healing process. Courteous neighbors assist the loser in making courageous new gains during recovery; insolent ones have the opposite effect. Parker had some good advice along these lines: "Eliminate resolutely from your life those people who are indifferent or hurtful to your feelings" (1981:78). Loss demands emotional resolutions which contribute to unity and wholeness. A neighbor's loss is like a house on fire; everyone ought to be willing to help put it out, but they don't. And that's the problem in providing adequate health care, for it takes everyone working closely together to provide quality health care.

Sympathy can help in providing health care, but it shouldn't stop there. For without perseverance, even a positive attitude toward the recipient is not enough, especially if the recipient does not respond in kind. Studies on aphasic adults have confirmed this insight. In extensive observations of 16 couples, Mulhall and Eisenson (1984:260) found that often the well spouse's sympathy turned to anger because the sick partner became more frustrated with their physical condition in response to the spouse's encouragement and attempts to help them. A predictable pattern was described: the well spouse showed sympathy which frustrated the aphasic spouse. This produced anger in the healthy spouse and caused depression in the aphasic spouse. In a follow-up study, Muller and Code (1984:269) realized that this inconsistency produced serious problems during the recovery process. They concluded that therapists should work more closely with the family in providing some realistic assessment about the outcome. It seems that the healthy mates were more optimistic about the condition of their mate than were the therapists. The problems compounded whenever the aphasic patient was the husband. The wife tended to be much more emotional about her problems: she cried, showed irritation, worried about the future. In other words, the wife had lost her security and protection, so she not only dealt with the problems of the husband, but also with her own insecurity.

The Necessity of Supporters

People live their lives inductively as they connect experiences together. These connections tend to take precedence over feelings and beliefs. Routine scheduling doesn't require much emotional input except in cases of emotional overload. However, that routine changes with a loss. Those with losses are left with a heightened state of emotionalism and sentimentality when habits are temporarily stripped away from the social fabric of their lives. During these times, people try to connect the "anchors" of experience with beliefs and sentiments. The result is that we give greater attention to other modes of comprehending our experiences; we may shift focus from the inductive (putting the parts of our lives into some logical whole) to the deductive frame of reference (wanting a meaningful and integrated whole from which to see it all). In addition to this shift in orientation, we are much more contemplative about life. That contemplativeness unleashes our imagination and opens us up to alternative considerations.

The shift in focus of attention is best understood by comparing Figure 8-3 with Figure 3-1 in Chapter 3. With a disruption in life, people experience change. They loose the emotional "anchors" of everyday habitual behaviors.

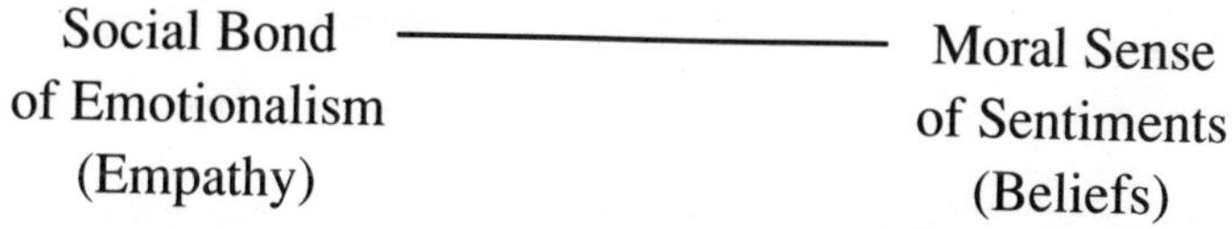

Figure 8-3. Heightened State of Loss.

In their place are left two floating aspects of human nature: the social bond of emotionalism and the moral sense of sentiments. Limited somewhat by the exploration of newness, they naturally look for some unified whole to regain an equilibrium in life. They find unification in several ways; various people— close friends, family, neighbors— give guidance and support to bridge the gap between the present and their former state. Supporters assist patients who find themselves in a state of dependence.

Before dependence, these patients lived independently. As loss set off the emotional alarm, these same patients responded promptly, but with increasing losses, routine patterns become disrupted. Patients may not even be able to solve their problems rationally or routinely. Emotions disrupt people; they then must deal with feelings of nervousness, anger, depression, and paranoia; other symptoms may include headaches, rapid heart beats, denial, and inability to concentrate. Fortunately, we have learned much about these patterns of emotions, and progress has been made in the management of stress.

While techniques and strategies for increasing emotion buffers occupy providers' minds, they should not forget the basics. What matters to patients, regardless of the intervention selected, is the support system around them. Ultimately, the effectiveness and efficiency of providers may not be measured by numbers of patients treated, or the kind of medical technology used. Nor does competitiveness in providing health care finally determine success. What finally matters is whether or not health care professionals are committed to providing emotional intervention along with everything else. Are they successful in caring for the emotions of others? Providers can assess their effectiveness by answering the following questions:

1) Have you been able to identify your feelings about the role of caregiving?
2) Have you recognized that you will probably feel isolated at times? Have you planned what you will do to combat that feeling? Can you say the same for anger? Depression? Guilt? Jealousy?
3) Have you ever felt proud of your ability to provide care for another person? Have you learned to savor those moments of tenderness and companionship that you and the recipient have shared? Do you remember to laugh at yourself and the situation (Horne, 1985:296)?

The following questions focus attention on the issues of providing support for an aging loved one; others could be asked about coping mechanisms:

1) Focus on what is, rather than on what is not, and stop

complaining to get sympathy or attention.

2) Give yourself a present of time, and while you are at it, do things to express your emotions.

3) Make time to participate in activities other than caregiving. Take time for other activities.

4) If you are depressed, do the hardest things first. Face your troubles as you are able to.

5) Train yourself to recognize your emotional signals. Stop what you are doing and attend to these emotional needs. It may mean just thirty seconds for some deep breathing (Hafen et al., 1982:16-17; Horne,1985:255).

Working at the University of Southern California in the field of gerontology, Zarit believes that caregivers should respond to practical and emotional demands. Fortunately, new technology makes the practical requirement easier to resolve: 1) Eating with special utensils and eating aids; 2) Mobility with access and ambulation aids such as ramps near doorways, crutches, canes, and even special bicycles; 3) Communication with hearing aids, computers, and bookholders, or letter boards, gestures, or pointing boards for those without verbal ability; 4) Independent living through environmental control using such items as powered wheelchairs, robots, electrical stimulation, and limb prosthetics. The ongoing development of computor and electronic technology has opened up whole new areas for the disabled and holds the promise for much improvement in the future (Childress, 1987:117-127).

Even after practical demands are met, the emotional demands still remain. They are special problems because "one important aspect of caregiving is its emotional burden...emotional pain..., and the tasks of caregiving can themselves be physically and emotionally exhausting" (Horne, 1985:xiv). It's the human electricity of emotions that presents the greatest challenge. As Marcel Prout put it: "The time which we have at our disposal every moment is elastic;

the passions that we feel expand it, those that we inspire contract it; and habit fills up what remains." Health care professionals intuitively know this, but they need reminding from time to time; they're humans with feelings just like their patients. Patients are told to be honest about their feelings—isolation, anger, depression, guilt, jealousy, fear, frustration, and joy; and providers need to be honest with themselves also. The ups and downs in emotions are what make people human, even though feelings come in a mixed package. "Sometimes it is bettersweet, and sometimes it is pure and rich and very exhilarating...to support each other, and if possible, share the experience of depending upon each other" (Horne,1985:254).

Chapter 9

Healthy Rediscovery of Dreams

One month after a horse ridding accident, Elle Becker wrote "I wish I were dead." Her accident caused not only a severe spinal cord injury, but also severe emotional depression. Indications of these feelings are seen in her notes while still at the hospital: "Hold me, and tell me I should not be afraid," or "non frustrated, sad, lonesome" (Becker 1987:12). She was an athletically inclined individual who suddenly had become a high-level paraplegic. In addition to the sudden life changes, the confinement, the depression and frustration; there were the negative labels associated with her condition. Elle was able to overcome those negative labels of "crippled, disabled, sexually inactive" as she discovered healthy dreams. Since that accident, she realized her dreams: to complete two degrees, write extensively, and counsel at the Kaiser Rehabilitation Center in Vallejo, California.

A dream combines people and treatment, normalization and integration, sociotechnical and personal satisfaction. "A motorized wheelchair and an electrical lift have freed my consciousness from such tedious concerns as getting around and going to the toilet independently; reduced architectural barriers in the community have made life much more pleasant also. They are greatly appreciated contributors to my Quality of Life (QOL)" (Vash, 1987:20). But the QOL changes along with realized dreams, so we must put on new dreams which are the hope of tomorrow. To reach present dreams is to rediscover the source of those earlier dreams.

According to Vash (1987:30), the number of those permanently limited by health conditions is increasing (37 percent) faster than the numbers being added to our total population (10 percent). Within those ranks are dreamers who seek creative ways to dream in spite of society's emphasis on wholeness and perfection. To not dream is easier, but necessity compels the dreamer. Healthy dreams and their realization require a host of actors and actresses. "Positive images, information and personal contact, cognitive dissonance, success models, positive associations, professional image creators, school experience, and medication can each prove powerful in attitude change" (Couch, 1987:52). Without healthy dreams, stereotypes continue, leaving "lingering fears, doubts, and even hostile attitude" (Yuker, 1979; Yunker and Block, 1987).

In spite of the odds against ever dreaming healthy dreams again, some of those who are recovering manage to do so. Vash (1987:11-12) found that "no difference between severely mobility-disabled and able-bodied groups exists in ratings of life satisfaction, or frustration with life." He found that "the majority accepted disablement as a fact of life. Only half used up a hypothetical 'one wish' on a surgery that would cure them." In a study that compared attitudes of providers with recipients, sexual impairment for men with spinal cord injuries ranked higher for staff than those affected. "Staff tended to overemphasize the importance of genital functioning." Loss of genital use in men with spinal cord injuries was labelled "terrible."

The patient needs reassurances about the future, desires become realized dreams through the norms of reciprocity. They are achieved by solving practical problems, and that takes team effort. Not all patients and their families realize how much healthy adjustment contributes to recovery. Objective medical analysis begins the treatment or recovery, but when combined with social empathy, families eliminate ambiguity about diagnosis, prognosis, and treatment courses. *Medical science begins recovery; sociology continues it.* In the process of struggling with losses, those who are recovering compensate for losses that may never be regained.

People evaluate handicaps, physical disabilities, illnesses, diseases, and health with different standards depending upon their definitions. If the public defines health as 1) general feeling about well-being, 2) absence of disease or pain, or 3) as the ability to perform in society, they may regard the handicapped with disdain. The injured person may also experience incongruities, the fallout of psychosocial emotions, from these social definitions. *That is where sympathetic others fill the gap and buffer the disabled from those less sensitive individuals in their environment.* "Emotional support is found in small, dense, close-knit networks; cognitive and material supports are more often found in large and loose-knit networks" (Jacobson, 1986:260).

Myocardial infarction patients are an example of one group of patients to whom emotional support is very important, since proper rehabilitation often demands significant life style adjustment. Research shows that these patients do not always comply, however. Miller et al. (1984) evaluated 141 cardiac patients during rehabilitation. All of the subjects were expected to modify their diets, take medications, stop smoking, increase physical activities, and reduce stress. The researchers found that compliance depended upon the the attitudes of patients, their perceptions of others' beliefs, original intentions, and ultimate behavior. Adherence to medical regimentation and successful completion depended upon the "perceived beliefs of significant others," a factor that proved to be even stronger than the patient's own beliefs. In fact, the patient's adherence to diet, smoking abstinence, exercise, medication, and control of stress correlated the highest with "perception of the significant other's belief" (1984:270).

To understand these social dynamics is to examine the stages in crises care, the importance of healthy dreams, the meaning of a breakthrough, the stages of recovery, the issues of multiple treatments, the necessity for changes in thinking and feeling, and the courage to be emotional. *These topics are social dimensions of emotions which buffer patients from the spiraling effects of a health crisis and make the difference in quality health care.*

Stages in Crises Care

Providers see patients in many settings: acute hospitalization, rehabilitation facilities, nursing home care, and home care.

Stages in crises care are predictable; as crisis and pain begin, providers treat systemic diseases and somatizatic disorder, "recurrent somatic symptoms for which there is no medical explanation" (Smith, 1986). Both the physical and emotional problems may continue into the second stage.

The second stage extends through relationships for treatment, then guidance through crises. First stage pains easily become second stage moods and generalized feelings. Providers devise treatments for body specific complaints, real or imagined, while also giving guidance. Doctors focus on the physical; therapists focus on self-care. Social workers attend to social matters; ministers comfort the grieving. This second stage of crisis integrates life: physical well-being, self-concepts, emotional stress, relationships, and fatigue.

If symptoms do not stop, then another transformation occurs. At this level emotions extend beyond the six senses, even beyond general feelings about lived experience. This third stage involves a higher dimension of collective consciousness. From health to illness, from illness to recovery, patients often publicly display anger over an injustice or about values. Patients evaluate social sentiments about handicaps or disabilities. Are these labels fair or just? In describing a particular case of a woman with Eisenmenger's syndrome, Napodano advocated that attending internists engage in "1) counseling, 2) joint decision making, 3) communication with all elements of her human support system, 4) learning about the legal and ethical issues relevant to her illness situation, and 5) identifying and using the most appropriate community services that may help her to achieve an acceptable level of independence, given the risks that exist" (1986:105).

"Doctoring and service to the sick transcend the diagnosis and treatment of diseases and the application of science and technology to the clinical context" (Napodano, 1986:122). Such suggestions are not new. Freud and Jung began with lower level sensations and feelings of the body only to establish psychoanalysis as a method of probing the mental dimensions. They discovered that deeply lodged feelings from pains and pleasures are rooted in biology, but that the method of analysis and treatment predetermined perceptions. Their epistemology (How do you know?) determined their ontology (What is really there?).

During Freud's era, people did not examine the association between symbolism (achievement motivation, goal setting, personal values) and behavior (health, life styles, illness). The diagnoses and treatments of Freud, therefore, were more biological. As one of his disciples, Jung explored the stream of consciousness whereby people collect myths, dreams, and ideas. These sentiments, which are deposited in human consciousness, remain in each generation. That consciousness forms the basis for values, priorities, and standards of behavior. Since it evolves collectively whenever people value their moral worth, consciousness is collectively expressed emotions. Few endorse this interpretation of emotions more so than Lifton. He believes that Jung combined the hope of earlier traditions with the "modern therapeutic ethos" (1979:16). Building on Jung's attempts, Lifton tries to synthesize opposites such as denial and affirmation, life and death. He believes that this synthesis is a necessity if people are ever to connect the "universal inner quest for continuous symbolic relationship to what has gone before and what will continue after our finite individual lives" (1979:17). Only with higher stages of symbolization, he thinks, will we ever connect the biological and historical stages of people.

Continuity and Change in Dreams

The symbolization of continuity and change applies to health care. It is natural that people strive for the continuity of life. Before crises, social thoughts are either based on those feelings which emerge from sense perception, or determined by generalized feelings which follow events and interruptions. Symbolization refers to how people connect themselves to various crises or traumatic events. After crises, people inevitably shift toward higher forms of symbolization. They are more serious about the future and meaning of life.

At the time of crises resulting from illness, accident, or loss, people initially stay in that basic mode of feeling related to sense perception. It is only later, after reflection, that these emotions shift towards higher forms. This process is understandably related to feelings after crisis. Low level feelings, along with early reflection about losses, begin at the point of impact. If there is bodily pain or injury, then that is where the focus of attention is. A shift in thinking inevitably occurs and emotions move toward higher levels of moral consciousness. It is then that people dream about life, goals, and relationships.

Lifton's elaboration of this process of striving for continuity has practical applications. This symbolization is a process whereby people integrate their lives when threatened with losses. In contrast to Lipton's symbolization, Crumbaugh et al. (1980) specify the dynamics of symbols and dreams. These dynamics revolve around things and encounters. Two questions identify them: What are the things recipients want to do now in light of their crisis? and Who are they doing them for? In analyzing emotions, these two dynamics relate significantly to a healthy recovery. In recovery, recipients have time for prolonged reflection about the meaning of life goals and relations. These two categories of goals and encounters are divided further. Goals are directed towards vocations, avocations, or causes. It is through these channels that people gain recognition and satisfaction in their accomplishments. What is it that when finished brings the greatest sense of satisfaction? Those dreams, and other issues, are reevaluated in the light of crisis,

In addition to goals, people organize their thinking around meaningful encounters and the sources of those encounters. Since crises and losses disrupt these relationships, these relationships must also be considered. Crumbaugh et al. (1980:83) use three relational subclasses as a practical guide in their work with recovering problem drinkers: subhuman, human, and superhuman. As the recipient evaluates the appropriateness of these relationships, their attention is diverted from the past into the future. This should aid them in working through the prolonged and often delayed responses to crisis which have disrupted meaningful patterns of interactions. It is in these encounters with pets (subhuman), people (human), or God (superhuman) that the emotional energy for recovery is found.

Since these relationships vary considerably, providers may not use all three subclasses. Some individuals value pets more than others do, and pets are a valuable resource for recovery of unstable emotions.   An advantage of pets is that they are not as threatening as people are, but pets lack the ability that people have to understand and accept "feelings of awe, hope, despair, desire" (1980:83). This quality of understanding and acceptance is especially important because crisis produces emotional strain which leads to feelings of isolation and loneliness.

The third relational subclass describes encounters with a higher power or God. Exactly what form and description this encounter takes varies. For some people it is an encounter with the ultimate Designer or force of the universe; for others, it is a personal God who forms the basis of their religious beliefs. The recipient can once again gain emotional strength and purpose from these encounters at a time when it is needed the most. Even though the encounter may be difficult to describe, if that encounter is meaningful, then it can be of value. "If you can sense in the worlds of telescope and microscope a glimpse of things felt but unseen; if you can grant on faith that there is some scheme of things, some sort of purpose and some kind of Being superior to man himself—then you have open to you, and in reality a far greater, source of existential encounter" (Crumbaugh, et al.,1980:97).

Loss comes unexpectedly, but it is vulnerability that distinguishes the prepared from the unprepared, and which divides people from their emotions. Salby and Glicksman (1985:3) list three distinctions in these dynamics. First, since the exact time of the crisis cannot be predicted, what distinguishes people is how they learn about and prepare for the unexpected. Second, since stability varies with the availability of resources, support filters out the vulnerable. Support is meaningful conversations, not just words. It takes time, requires attention, separates topics, reveals uncertainties, and uncovers feelings. Meaningful conversations direct the release of emotions,the balance of budgets, and the actions of friends.

Third, since crises tests values, people reevaluate their priorities in the chill and stupor of loss. Anne Frank wrote in her diary: "I can shake off everything if I write. My sorrows disappear, my courage is reborn...I can recapture everything when I write—my thoughts, my ideas, my fantasies." The reevaluation can even extend to beliefs about survival itself. Tragedies rule people, people do not rule tragedies. Tragedies affect people's physical well-being. So what people look for is not a rehearsing of the old way, but a discovery of something new; they look for a breakthrough, medically and socially.

A Breakthrough

Recipients of health care work through several deliberations: What to do next? and What relationships are important now? These questions form the basis for healthy recovery. Through this guided design, providers interact with recipients about their dreams and future plans. This process of interaction is surprisingly similar to the one advocated by Jung; he believed that a breakthrough in struggles comes only as people connect their dreams with the great truths of life. Jung saw emotions as the vehicle which transported people from "darkness into light." Without transformations, dreams remain in darkness (Hughes, 1959:199):

What happens to a dream deferred?
Does it dry up?
Or fester like a sore and then run?

Does it stink like rotten meat?
Or crust and sugar over,
Like a syrupy sweet?

Maybe it just sags,
Like a heavy load.
Or does it explode?

Following a crisis, transformations answer the need to propel dreams into reality. Jung advocated a type of social emotive analysis and therapy to adequately utilize this emotional energy. He encouraged his patients in therapy to describe their dreams, and he then interpreted the social context of those dreams for the purpose of propelling the dreams along as "bottled up emotions" needing an outlet, or as "stored up energy" seeking an object. Jung evaluated the dismantling of social sentiments in a more serious light than Freud did. In a broader sense, Jung did not forget the idealistic (mystical religious experience) and the role that emotions play in determining and achieving a "spiritual destiny." This type of approach was obviously less scientific than Freud's, yet Jung emphasized an intervention of emotions surprisingly close to the ones currently recommended (see section on Multimodality). For Jung, therapy uncovers meaning and purpose in life; it preserves traditions and religion. To do away with religious beliefs drastically alters society because these beliefs, in contrast with narrowly direct and objective knowledge, comprise the indirect, subjective wisdom of collective emotions accumulated over time.

Society's loss of these traditions, along with it's loss of individuals, restricts alternatives for action. Whether people use these alternatives or not is their choice, but they give recipients who value historic time another valuable resource to cope with the stress of emotions over time. Because severe losses leave irreparable damage, recipients desire a breakthrough in time. They know that time is inelastically distributed, not expandable for anyone, regardless of their wealth or status. But recipients also know that time provides opportunities for people to fulfill dreams, but that losses shatter them into a thousand pieces.

Some losses are like the nursery rhyme: "All the kings horses and all the kings men can't put Humpty back together again." Loss of control in life can give way to hopelessness. The 5th century Greek philosopher Sophocles said that "time eases all things." Is this true? Are the hindsights of traditions and beliefs more valuable in hopeless cases than scientific predictions of survival rates? Does historic time broaden the frame of reference much like old family portraits do? When individuals look back over time, can they see more clearly and objectively what happened to them in time and how that incident continues its effects? Figure 9-1 diagrams the sensation of pain and the response of sentiments.

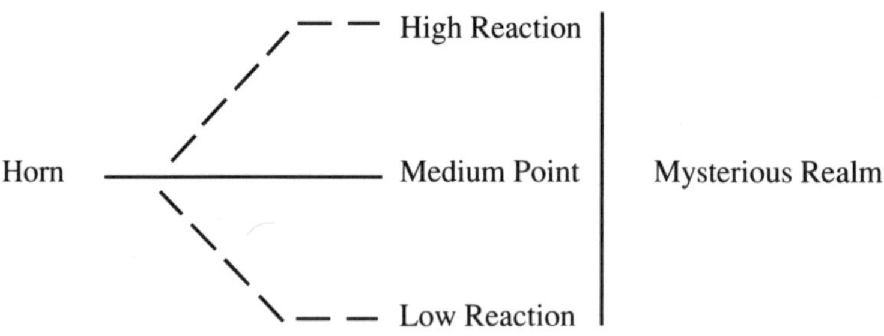

Figure 9-1. The Sentiments of Emotions.

When the horns of hopelessness sound, their intensity is deeply felt. The body responds with an irregular fluctuation, depending upon how long the horn blasts last. Even with short blasts, people are sandwiched between emotions and sensations pushing and pulling with each heart beat. Subjective body sensations are experienced; objective body signs are evaluated. Then selves (providers) evaluate selves (recipients) using a variety of methods. People finally confront the mysterious realm where they, like the 17th century poet, might ask questions about these sensations and life itself (Brook, 1983:257):

> What is this life: A frenzy, an illusion,
> A shadow, a delirium, a fiction.
> The greatest good's but little, and this life
> Is but a dream, and dreams are only dreams.

Stages of Recovery

These insights can be applied to uncover the stages of crisis management and recovery (Broadwell, 1987). For this to happen, however, providers and recipients should form partnerships in quality care. Face-to-face interaction (Figure 9-2) works best in positive, caring relationships.

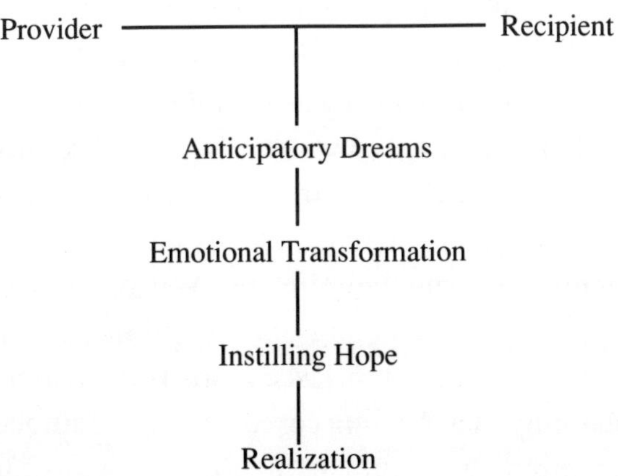

Figure 9-2. The Growth of Recovery.

This is where nonverbal and emotional communication occurs, where we find "empathy, warmth, self-confidence, expertness, active participation, and the ability to convey hope" (Slaikeu, 1984:301). In environments conducive for growth, recipients "will be open and expressive about their feelings" (Slaikeu,1984:301). The "anticipatory dreams" in Figure 9-2 is a concept taken from current techniques of intervention: guided self dialogue, idealized self-image technique, and a gestalt therapy known as the empty chair. The first of these allows the client to replace negative thoughts or ideas with positive ones, while the other two techniques encourage the client to dream about the future. Theraptists assume that positive images become reality over time, but only as recipients engage themselves in imaginary dialogues. The Gestaldt procedure was developed by Fritz Perls (Slaikeu,1984:301); clients sit in one chair while facing an empty chair. Clients then talk to themselves about their feelings, beliefs, and attitudes by switching from one chair to another.

Anticipatory dreaming is followed by emotional transformation (Figure 9-2). Patients reflect on their future and then take ownership of their dreams. Providers encourage the emotional transformation of their patients so that they can convert their emotional energy into positive action. A provider "communicates understanding and empathy by reformulating and summarizing the client's explicit statements, by attending to and commenting on the client's nonverbal or paraverbal signals" (Slaikeu, 1984:295). Unless given the mandate to decide for patients, providers should allow patients to pursue their dreams (Wilson,1986). The focus is on present perceptions, feelings, and flexibility to adjust to social environments (Belkin, 1986:194). Hope is the patient's "estimate of the probability of achieving certain goals" (Campbell, 1987:19). That is why providers should instill hope that goals can be realized. Otherwise, patients will be negative about the future, sense that they can do little to change it, become passive, and exhibit negative emotions. "By focusing on reducing the sources of a patient's hopelessness, the professional may be able to alleviate crises more effectively" (Campbell, 1987:21). Once dreams are firmly planted, they begin to grow until they become publicly visible. What begins as small seeds of possibility, known to a few, gradually evolves into the next stage of realization. Possibilities become realities when recipients move into action and realize their dreams.

Multimodality

Emotional engagement and transformation (provider to recipient) produce the vital dynamics of health recovery. Yalom has documented their importance in group intervention strategies. Based on his clinical research, group support does inspire and motivate recipients in times of hopelessness. Inspiration comes through strong emotional support wherever the recipient: 1) feels that they can really change, 2) knows that they are not alone, 3) sees that they are important to someone else, 4) understands that someone else is important to them, and 5) accepts their feelings of frustration during the whole process. Yalom's findings indicate that inspiration involves: installation of hope, universality, altruism, cohesiveness, and catharsis.

Motivation is also enhanced through positive group interaction, assuming that other curative factors are also present. Researchers have identified at least five characteristics that motivate recipients to action. Patients respond appropriately by: 1) relearning where needed, 2) learning to get along with others, 3) watching others, 4) overcoming self-defeating misconceptions, and 5) living their own lives. Groups are the mediating factors as patients progress in the following areas: corrective recapitulation, development of social skills, imitative behavior, interpersonal learning, and existential factors (Kendall,1984:540-543).

These multimodalies are techniques which suggest that either positive or negative emotions have a profound effect on the recovery of patients. Since people communicate emotionally and rationally, both types of communication may motivate recipients as they cope with and recover from their crises (Table 9-1).

Table 9-1. The Content and Process of Coping and Recovering

Content	Process
Tactics & Strategies for Coping	Obtaining Information for Cognitive Rational Therapy
Meaning & Purpose for Living	Discovering Dreams for Social Emotive Therapy
Reorienting and Reintroduction into Society	Establishing Equilibrium

Table 9-1 combines rational and emotive functions, and is a framework for understanding the dynamics of healthy recovery. Through intervention (process and content of interacting), providers skillfully engage recipients in at least three activities (the rows). Providers use tactics and strategies for obtaining objective information about coping with change, necessary information for solving problems and making decisions. Next is meaning and purpose for living. Whether providers actually do this or not is irrelevant, and even if health providers are involved in discovery dreams, many of these remain private in nature. These are valuable resources that lead to the third listing under content in Table 9-1, reorientation and reintroduction into society. These work as a process to help the patient reestablish an equilibrium within society.

Changes in Thinking and Feeling

There are only three options in a difficult situation. One option is to move away or leave that environment. People hope that they will cope better in a new environment. If this option is not desirable or possible, then a second option is to change the situation, make it more acceptable. Rosellini and Worden (1985) suggest that to change situations requires asking these four questions: 1) What am I feeling? 2) Why am I feeling this way? 3) What can I do about it? and 4) What am I going to do about it? This particular process, or one like it, forces patients to not only deal with their emotions, but also the sources of those frustrations. The grief process (recognizing emotions and expressing them) helps recipients focus on solutions to change the situation.

There is still a third option: to accept the situation as it is. This option is available when it is not possible to leave or to change the person, place, thing, experience, or condition that is causing the problem. This involves changing one's thoughts and feelings about what has happened. Even though radical changes in thinking and feeling only occur with considerable struggle or a devastating crisis, it is possible to act in spite of these struggles. Patients who emotionally accept undesirable health situations must still seek solutions to their problems of adjustment and acceptance of things as they are. It might help to evaluate the problem/solutions from the perspectives of responsibilities, roles, and relationships. Solutions to problems depend upon whether people accept the responsibility to work together. For example, those discharged from acute care settings and their family members must adjust in several ways. Patients and families accept responsibility for on-going care by understanding their roles and working together to get everything accomplished. The dynamics of problem/solution, change/adjustment are often overlooked as providers prepare patients for release. Having a plan of action should assist patients and their families in making these adjustments (Blazyk and Canavan, 1986). The three dimensions of change allow patients to see both near and distant problems, and to see practical solutions for healthy recovery (Table 9-1).

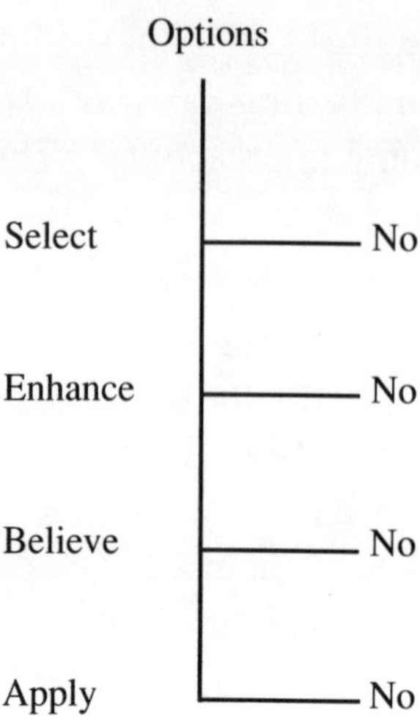

Figure 9-3. A Flow Chart for Healthy Recovery.

Figure 9-3 shows how the process of recovery works. An underlying assumption is that others are the significant factors in making it work—both the patient and the support group. Selecting all the relevant information and knowing all the options obviously are important. In consultation with the medical staff, supporters encourage patients in healthy recovery, thus enhancing their efforts. Patients either believe in their decisions and want to recover or they don't. It appears that the bonds of relationships directly affect dynamics, positively or negatively. Wethington and Kessler found that perceived support—not necessarily the received support— seems to be the critical factor in adjustment to stressful life events (1986:78-89). Part of the debate about social supporters and the mechanism of support centers around the ways that this support is transferred to recipients. Based on the findings of Wethington and Kessler, even the perception of help makes a difference. Actually, help in practical ways does matter, but even the perception of help without any of it forthcoming seems to make adjustment smoother.

The last step in Figure 9-3 is applying the other steps. Patients must build these insights and strategies into habits and life styles.

Courage to be Emotional

Not all people want to be emotional, especially if they suffer intense emotional feelings. When researchers asked a group of chemically dependent patients what one person they desired most to be like, approximately 80 percent of them answered "Mr. Spock," from the TV series Startrek. When asked why they chose him, they said that Mr. Spock responds to crisis quite calmly, without any emotional gyration. They also said that Captain Kirk— like the rest of us—struggles, feels, weeps, cries, agonizes, and most of all, hurts emotionally. Rosellini and Worden appropriately label this the "Spock Syndrome: Born Vulcan" (1985:20).

Yes, life would be easier for if we weren't so emotional; if we were like Spock, above and beyond emotional outbursts and pain. But that isn't the way it is, and Roselline and Worden found that unrecognized emotions in the form of anger keeps their clients and their families from achieving recovery. Rosellini and Worden ask their clients to take an emotional inventory by answering some basic questions about their feelings. The following six questions have been adopted for our own purposes:

1. Do we accept our emotions as natural and normal expressions?
2. When recovering from health problems, do we take our feelings into account?
3. Can we emotionally accept the changes since our health crisis?
4. Do we accept our feelings without guilt or shame?
5. Can we live with our emotional baggage long after health care?
6. Can we cope with a variety of emotional expressions both intense or mild?

To answer yes for each or most of these six questions requires courage and acceptance of our humanness. The way we handle our feelings has much to do with the rediscovery of dreams. Pearsall lists ten ways to develop healthier emotions and lifestyles: learn to laugh, covet loving relations, simplify your life, accept your physical conditions, visit the doctor, be optimistic, take charge of your life each day, stay calm even under stress, be grateful for being alive, and set priorities (1987). Emotions give vitality to life "through emotionality, sympathy, violence, fellow-feeling, shared emotionality, emotional footings, and emotional presentations of self "(Denzin, 1984:278). As people draw others into their lives, they become more than machines or Vulcans like Spock. Emotions give "the everyday world and the ordinary people who live in that world a sense of joy, bewilderment, pain, confusion, satisfaction, and pleasure that no other form of conduct can" (Denzin,1984:278).

People reconstruct meaning in crises through emotions, but it takes courage to be human and emotional. Effectiveness and efficiency, characteristics of our bureaucratic institutions, obstruct emotional expressions. So rather than express their true feelings, people learn to manage or even suppress them. The social norms often dictate what people say and how they express their feelings; the gap between true feelings and artificial presentation widens. That does not mean, according to Erich Fromm, that people should ever stop feeling, longing, or dreaming about a "world in which love, freedom, and justice are rooted.... Only a changed social reality, a society that realizes the principles of love and human autonomy throughout its structure, can satisfy this demand" (Funk,1982:294-295).

But we don't have to wait for changes in the whole of society before we act in our hospitals. An emotional crisis or loss is the ideal opportunity to encourage the expression of emotions. Health care providers must incorporate both stress management for emotional overload and practical sensitivity by sympathetic listening. Without any neglect of traditional medical requirements, professionals could also orient their skills towards the emotional side of health care. Otherwise, emotional exhaustion and loss of emotional energy make it all the more difficult for patients to act courageously. Patients would be less likely to get bogged down in unhealthy attitudes if they had the ability to understand the crisis, disclose their feelings, assess their coping abilities, and resolve conflict and realize their potential for emotional stamina.

Each one of us takes a view of life that makes it either impossible to accept gratefully a gain or imperative to endure persistently a loss. One is oriented to now; the other to later. One gets; the other gives. Neither, however, avoids loss, and both respond emotionally. How else can we explain a case where one is never satisfied in getting; the other is always satisfied in giving, even in losses. Some recipients respond to gains with ingratitude, others to losses with gratitude to God. Crises in life may not force us to ultimate meaning and priorities so much as they bring out what a person's meaning and purpose in life is. In experiences of loss, people sort out a variety of issues, and "the questions of ultimate meaning and the significance of the individual are written large" (Schoenberg and Preston,1983:166).

Beliefs and persuasions about the future make up the ability to dream about something beyond our present experiences. Religious beliefs also become a crucial factor in handling these types of crises. These beliefs remain intact during recovery when practical matters come into play with group intervention strategies. Gatherings of a natural group play an important role for everyone as they sense what others are feeling. There must be an active rather than passive approach to these events, for only then are people able to counter "feelings of isolation, abandonment, and guilt; and decrease feelings of helplessness and low self-esteem" (1982:278).

Servan-Schreiber describes affect as the black box "which is little known, badly managed, and therefore gives us constant trouble" (1987:90). The content of emotions does vary: humor, grief, desires, passions, courage. It is the courage that allows us to live better. To be courageous is to follow the example of others who survive; others who aren't possessed with the problems; who shift their attention toward other activities; who see life as a whole; who plan for difficulties; who face problems; who know their limitations; who solve the source of problems; who aren't slaves to what others think; who are flexible; and who combine work with play (1987:110-112). To be courageous is "to face up to the idea of our death and to find our individual means of accepting it" (Servan-Schreiber, 1987:138). It is to be ourselves; it is to accept what cannot be changed.

Summary and Conclusion

The contrasting emotions experienced in health settings do not flow from biology alone; nor from the psyche alone; nor from the prolonged suffering alone; nor from responses of family alone, but from social events which fulfill and transcend the immediate health care setting. These are social events which somehow link people to those living and to those not yet born.

The broader topic is quality health care and service; the emotions of those providing and those receiving; the conditions which promote a climate for emotional stability. Stressful situations that involve clients, family, friends, or associates inevitably create emotions that are normal, erratic, and intense. If properly understood, effectively dealt with, and finally released, these emotions can be important factors in maintaining or reestablishing an emotional equilibrium. However, most people do not validate or release the emotions that surround these encounters. Patients cope not only with outside events (difficulties, restrictions, obstacles), but also with inside emotions. Events produce a full range of emotions from love to hate, anxiety to apprehension, and from hopelessness to exhaustion. Regardless of how people handle their emotions, others are also involved.

The systems of interaction are the body-mind emotions. Patients may interact with the hospital staff (organization), their families (group), and the patient-community system (Viney and

Clark, 1986). Health care is a system of community relationships in which people cope with the emotions of situations (Denzin,1984). But that community extends beyond physical proximity. It is the bonding of family, providers, and friends as they interact, regardless of physical proximity. This intensely cohesive factor emerges from affectivity, but extends beyond to quality and satisfaction with services rendered. It is labor intensive and emotionally draining. Since the management of emotional stress requires special skills, and since the equilibrium for emotional balance is often tilted toward strained relations, the study of emotions warrants continued scientific investigation.

That research must go beyond the routine and consider the following characteristics: interactive, social, and emotive. Researchers should investigate what others do not: the examination of how emotions are distributed in the social network of relations between recipient and provider. But the research questions should be even more specific than that: What social factors contribute to higher levels of anxiety in the care of the sick? For if we know the answer to that question, then providers can not only increase their effectiveness and efficiency of services, but *they can also discover the "buffers" to cope with the emotional baggage that those services produce.*

This text is concerned with the *buffer of emotions* and the proper place of emotions both in the sickness of patients and in the care given by professionals. Emotions are found everywhere in our society, but especially in medical and health crises. During these times emotions are naturally directed towards incidents, others, self, and God.

Since the direction of emotions is subjectively expressed by feelings, and since those feelings vary somewhat illogically, quality care establishes stability of emotions. Because of their erratic nature, emotions must be balanced against reason, but at the same time let us not isolate feelings from thoughts, or science from art, or patients from the personal touch of professionals. Instead let us unite our resources as they are united in the experiences of life, where the interpretations come from both factual denotations and emotional connotations. After all, the real issue is not whether reason is preferred over emotions, but whether both contribute to quality health care. It is not likely that we will achieve quality health care until we start balancing the importance of medical competence against the compassion of professional sensitivity.

Quality care comes from several sources: common sense and correct decisions. Philosophically speaking, "losing is the price we pay for living. It is also the source of much of our growth. Making our way from birth to death, we also have to make our way through the pain of giving up some portion of what we cherish. We have to deal with our necessary losses" (Viorst, 1986). From a sociological viewpoint, caring professionals are the source of that quality care. At the American Management Association's 57th Conference, Frederick I. Herzberg spoke of passiveness and apathy within the ranks of professional managers. He challenged providers to adopt this creed: "Passion for life's purpose and compassion for life's betrayals." Quality care lies within our grasp: "Our fate is in our hands. The uncertainties are not in knowing what to do, not in science, not in economics. The uncertainties lie in our ability to discipline ourselves and our individual and collective wills to act with courage and compassion in a host of forums, from the Congress, state legislatures, city halls, school boards, hospital and corporate boardrooms, union halls to doctors' offices, and our own homes" (Califano, 1986:225).

Bibliography

Adelmann, Pam. "Freshening Freud for Us All." Detroit Free Press, 13 Sept. 1987.

Ahearn, Frederick L. and Raquel E. Cohen, eds. Disasters and Mental Health: An Annotated Bibliography. Rockville, Maryland: U.S. Department of Health and Human Services, 1984.

Alexy, Betty. "Goal Setting and Health Risk Reduction." Nursing Research 34 (1985):283-288.

Anastas, Lila L. How to Stay Out of the Hospital: A Practical Guide to Healthy Options and Alternatives. Emmaus, Pennsylvania: Rodale Press, 1986.

Association of American Medical Colleges. Physicians for the Twenty-First Century. Washington, D.C.: AAMC, 1984.

Atkinson, Thomas , Ramsay Liem, Joan H. Liem. "The Social Costs of Unemployment: Implications for Social Support." Journal of Health and Social Behavior 27 (1986):317-331.

Barker, Philip. Using Metaphors in Psychotherapy. New York: Brunner, 1985.

Barton, A. H. Communities in Disaster. Garden City, New York: Doubleday, 1969.

Batson, C. Daniel and Jay S. Coke. "Empathic Motivation of Helping Behavior." Social Psychophysiology. eds. John T. Cacioppo and Richard E. Petty. New York: The Guilford Press. 1983. 417-433.

Becker, Elle Friedman. "The Paraplegic: The Story of Elle." Interdisciplinary Rehabilitation in Trauma. eds. John J. Gerhardt, Echkhart Reiner, Bernd Schwaiger, and Philip King. Baltimore: Williams and Wilkins, 1987: 10-21.

Becker, Ernest. The Denial of Death. New York: The Free Press, 1975.

Belkin, Gary S. Contemporary Psychotherapies. Monterey, California:Brooks/ Cole Publishing Company, 1987.

Berdine, William H. and A. Edward Blackhurst, eds. An Introduction to Special Education. 2nd. ed. New York: Little Brown, 1985.

Berg, Ellen. "New Sections Probe Emotions and Culture." Footnotes (1987): 1-3.

Berg, M. "Patient Education and the Physician-Patient Relationship." Journal of Family Practice 24 (1987):169-171.

Bergsma, Jurrit and David C. Thomasma. Health Care: Its Psychosocial Dimensions. Pittsburgh, Pennsylvania: Duquesne U. Press. 1982

Blazyk S. and M. M. Canavan. "Managing the Discharge Crisis Following Catastrophic Illness or Injury." Social Work Health Care 11 (1986):19-32.

Bloch, Signey and Eric Crouch. Therapeutic Factors in Group Psychotherapy. Oxford: Oxford U. Press, 1985.

Bloom, Samuel. "Institutional Trends in Medical Sociology." Journal of Health and Social Behavior 27 (1986):265-276.

Bloomfield, Harold H. and Robert B. Kory. Health and Happiness. New York: Simon and Schuster, 1978.

Bolton, Robert and Dorothy Grover Bolton. Social Style/Management Style. New York: American Management Associations, 1984.

Bosse, Raymond and Charles L. Rose. Smoking and Aging. Lexington, Massachusetts:Lexington Books, 1984.

Boyle, Coleen A. "Postservice Mortality Among Vietnam Veterans." Journal of American Medical Association 257 (1987):790-795.

Bozarth-Campbell, Alla. Life Is Goodby, Life Is Hello: Grieving Well Through All Kinds of Loss. Minneapolis, Minnesota: Comp Care Publication, 1986.

Bramwell, Lillian and Ann L. Whall. "Effect of Role Clarity and Empathy on Support Performance and Anxiety." Nursing Research 35 (1986): 282-287.

Breedlove, Charlene. "Osleriana." Journal of American Medical Association 257 (1987) 467.

Brooks, Stephen. The Oxford Book of Dreams. Oxford: Oxford U. Press, 1983.

Brown, Barbara B. Between Health and Illness. New York: Bantam Books, 1985.

Brown, Marie Annette. "Social Support During Pregnancy: A Unidimensional or A Multidimensional Construct." Nursing Research 35 1986): 4-9.

Brown, Roger. Social Psychology. 2nd ed. New York: Free Press, 1986.

Buck, Ross. The Communication of Emotion. New York: The Guilford Press, 1984.

Cacioppo, John T. and Richard E. Petty, eds. Social Psychophysiology. New York: The Guilford Press, 1983.

Calhoun, Cheshire and Robert C. Solomon. What is an Emotion? New York: Oxford U. Press, 1984.

Califano, Joseph A. America's Health Care Revolution: Who Lives? Who Dies? Who Pays? New York: Random House, 1986.

Campbell, Linda. "Hopelessness." Journal of Psychosocial Nursing 25 (1987):18-22.

Cancian, Francesca and Steven Gardon. "Content Analysis of Love and Anger." Paper at American Sociological Association, 1986.

Canavan-Gumpert, Donna, Katherine Garner and Peter Gumpert. The Success-Fearing Personality. Lexington,Massachusetts: Lexington Books, 1978.

Centers for Disease Control. "Postservice Mortality Among Vietnam Veterans." Journal for American Medical Association 257 (1987):790-795.

Childress, Dudley S. "Rehabilitation Engineering and Technology: The Right Tech." Public Policy Issues Impacting the Future of Rehabilitation in America. ed., William G. Emener. Stillwater, Oklahoma: National Clearing House of Rehabilitation Training Materials, 1987:112-130

Clark, Carolyn Chambers. Wellness Nursing: Concepts, Theory, Research, and Practice. New York: Springer Publishing Company, 1986.

Cobb, S. and S. Kasl. Termination—the Consequences of Job Loss. Cincinnati, Ohio: U. S. Department of Health Education and Welfare, 1977.

Cohen, Jerome, Joseph W. Cullen, and L. Robert Martin, eds. Psychosocial Aspects of Cancer. New York: Raven Press, 1982.

Cohen, Sheldon and Karen Matthews. "Social Support, Type A Behavior and Coronary Artery Disease." Behavior and Psychosomatic Medicine 49 (1987): 325-330.

Condon, John T. "Psychological Disability in Women Who Relinquish a Baby for Adoption." Medical Journal of Australia 144 (1986):117-119.

Couch, Robert H. "Societal Attitudes Related to Services for People with Disabilities." Public Policy Issues Impacting the Future of Rehabilitation in America. ed., William G. Emener. Stillwater, Oklahoma: National Clearing House of Rehabilitation Training Materials, 1987: 112-130.

Cousins, Norman. "The Anatomy of An Illness." New England Journal of Medicine 295 (1976):1458-1463.

The Healing Heart. New York: Avon Printing, 1984.

Crumbaugh, James C., William M. Wood, and W. Chadwick Wood. Logotherapy New Help for Problem Drinkers. Chicago: Nelson-Hall, 1980.

Darley, Frederic L. Aphasia. Philadelphia: W. B. Saunders Company, 1982.

Dawson, Carolyn. "Hypertension, Perceived Clinician Empathy, and Patient Self Disclosure." Research in Nursing and Health 8 (1986):191-198.

Denzin, Norman K. On Understanding Emotion. New York: Jossey-Bass 1984.

DeVon, Holli and Marjorie J. Powers. "Health Beliefs, Adjustment to Illness, and Control of Hypertension." Research in Nursing and Health (1986): 10-16.

DiMatteo, Robin M., Louise M. Prince, and Ron Hays. "Nonverbal Communication in the Medical Context: The Physician-Patient Relationship." Nonverbal Communication in the Clinical Context. eds. Peter David Blanck, Ross Buck, and Robert Rosenthal. The University Park, Pennsylvania: Pennsylvania State U. Press, 1986:74-98.

Dohrewend, Barbara S. and Bruce D. Dohrewend. Stressful Life Events: Their Nature and Effects. New York: Wiley, 1974.

Doi, Tokeo. The Anatomy of Dependence. Tokyo: Kodansha Press, 1982.

Duck, Steve. Human Relationships: An Introduction to Social Psychology. Beverly Hills, California: Sage Publications, 1986.

Dugger, James G. The New Professional:An Introduction for the Human Services Worker. 2nd ed. Monterey, California:Brooks/Cole Publishing, 1980.

Eells, Mary Ann Walsh. "Interventions with Alcoholics and Their Families." Nursing Clinics of North America 21 (1986):493-504.

Eisenberg, Nancy. Altruistic Emotion, Cognition, and Behavior. Hillsdale, New Jersey: Lawrence Erlbaum Associates, 1986.

Eisenson, Jon. Adult Aphasia. 2nd ed. Englewood Cliffs, New Jersey: Prentice Hall, 1984.

Engel, Frema and Shirley Marsh. "Helping the Employee Victim of Violence in Hospitals." Community Psychiatry 37 (1986):159-162.

Entralgo, Pedro Lain. "What Does the Word Good Mean in Good Patient?" Changing Values in Medicine. Cornell U. Medical College: University Publications of America, 1979:127-143.

Erikson, K. T. "Loss of Community at Buffalo Creek." American Journal of Psychiatry 133 (1976):302-305.

Eyer, Joseph. "Hypertension as a Disease of Modern Society." Stress and Survival. ed. Charles A. Garfield. St. Louis: C. V. Mosby Company, 1979.

Feuerstein, Michael, Elise E. Labbe and Andrzej R. Kuczmierczyk. Health Psychology: A Psychobiological Perspective. New York: Plenum Press, 1986.

Fox, Peter D. and Willis B. Goldbeck. Health Care Cost Management: Private Sector Initiatives. Ann Arbor, Michigan:Health Administration Press, 1984.

Frank, Jerome D. "Nuclear Death: An Unprecedented Challenge to Psychia- try and Religion." The American Journal of Psychiatry 141 (1984): 1342-1348.

Freeman, Howard E., Sol Levine, and Leo G. Reeder. Handbook of Medical Sociology. Englewood Cliffs: Prentice-Hall, 1979.

Fritz, Wanona S. "Maintaining Wellness: Yours and Theirs." Nursing Clinics of North America 19 (1984):263-269.

Funk, Rainer. Eric Fromm: The Courage to be Human. New York: Contin-uum, 1982.

Garfield, Charles A. Stress and Survival: The Emotional Realities of Life-Threatening Illness. St. Louis: C.V. Mosby Company, 1979.

Gaylin, Willard. Rediscovering Love. New York: Viking, 1986.

Gazda, George M., William C. Childers, and Richard P. Walters. Interper-sonal Communication: A Handbook for Health Professionals. Rockville, Maryland: Aspen Publication, 1982.

Gelles, Richard J. "Family Violence." Annual Review of Sociology. eds. Ralph H. Turner and James F. Short. Vol. 11. Palo Alto, California: Annual Reviews Inc., 1985.

Gibbs, J. R. "Defensive Communication." The Journal of Communications 3 (1961): 141-148

Given, Charles W., Barbara A. Given, and Bryan W. Coyle. "Prediction of Patient Attrition From Experimental Behavioral Interventions." Nursing Research 34 (1985):299.

Golden J. Golden, Sandra S. Alcaparras, Fred D. Strider and Benjamin Graber, eds. Applied Techniques in Behavior Medicine. New York: Grune and Stratton, 1981.

Goldberg, Evelyn, Pearl Van Natta and George W. Comstock. "Depressive Symptoms, Social Networks and Social Support of Elderly Women." American Journal of Epidemiology 121 (1985): 448-456.

Goodwin, Donald W. Anxiety. New York: Ballantine, 1982.

Gordon, James S. "Alternative Services and Mental Health." Therapeutic Intervention:Healing Strategies for Human Services. eds. Uri Rueveni, Ross V. Speck, and Joan L. Speck. New York: Human Science Press, 1982:19-32.

Greer, William R. "The Rapidly Changing Health-Care Industry." The New York Times, September 1986: 52.

Hafen, Brent Q., Brenda Peterson, and Kathryn J. Frandsen. The Crisis Intervention Handbook. Englewood Cliffs, New Jersey: Prentice-Hall, 1982.

Hall, James A. Interpretation of Jungian Dreams. Toronto Canada: Inner City Books, 1983.

Hansell, N. The Person in Distress. New York: Human Sciences Press, 1976.

Hansen, James C. Clinical Implications of the Family Life Cycle. Rockville, Maryland: Aspen Publication, 1983.

Hargreaves, A. C., G. I. Krell, B. Blakeney and Ryan M. Blizzard. "Dealing With Disaster." American Journal of Nursing 79 (1979):268-271.

Harrigan, J. A. and R. Rosenthal. "Self Touching and Impressions of Others." Personality and Social Psychology 13 (1987):492-512.

Hartsough, Don M. "Planning for Disaster: A New Community Outreach Program for Mental Health Centers. Journal of Community Psychology 10 (1982):255-264.

Hartsough, Don M. and Diane Garaventa Myers. Disaster Work and Mental Health: Prevention and Control of Stress Among Workers. Rockville, Maryland: National Institutes of Mental Health, 1985.

Hays, David and C.E. Ross. "The Effects of Exercise, Overweight, and Physician Health." Journal of Health and Social Behavior 27 (1986): 387-400.

Henderson, George and Willie V. Bryan. Psychosocial Aspects of Disability. Springfield, Illinois: Charles C Thomas, 1984.

Hendin, Herbert and Ann Pollinger Haas. "Combat Adaptations of Vietnam Veterans Without Posttraumatic Stress Disorders." American Journal of Psychiatry 141 (1984):956-960.

Hilfiker, David. Healing the Wounds: A Physician Looks at His Work. New York: Pantheon Books, 1985.

Hill, R. "Generic Features of Families Under Stress." Crisis Intervention: Selected Readings. ed. H. N. Parad. New York: Family Service Association of America, 1965.

Hine, Frederick R., Robert C. Carson, George L. Maddox, Robert J. Thompson, Jr.and Redford B. Williams, Jr. Introduction to Behavioral Science in Medicine. New York: Springer-Verlag, 1985.

Hochschild, Arlie R. The Managed Heart: Commercialization of Human Feelings. Berkeley: U. of California Press, 1983.

Hoff, Lee Ann. People in Crisis: Understanding and Helping. 2nd ed. Reading, Massachusetts: Addison-Wesley Publishing, 1984.

Holmes, Thomas H. and Richard H. Rahe. "The Social Readjustment Rating Scale." Journal of Psychosomatic Research 11 (1967):213-218.

Homans, Peter. Jung in Context. Chicago: The U. of Chicago Press, 1979.

Horne, Jo. Care Giving: Helping An Aging Loved One. Glenview, Illinois: Lifelong Learning Division, 1985.

Howard, George, Don W. Nance, and Pennie Myers. Adaptive counseling and Therapy: A Systematic Approach to Selecting Effective Treatments. San Francisco: Jossey-Bass Publishers, 1987.

Hughes, Langston. "Harlem," The Panther and the Lash. Selected Poems of Langston Hughes. New York: Alfred A. Knopf, 1959.

Jack, Lynette W. "Using Play in Psychiatric Rehabilitation." Journal of Psychosocial Nursing 25 (1987):17-20.

Jackson, Edgar N. Coping With The Crisis in Your Life. Northvale, New Jersey: Jason Arronson, 1983.

Jacobson, David E. "Types of Training of Social Support." Journal of Health and Social Behavior 27 (1986):250-264.

Jacobson, G. R. and D. Lindsay. "Screening of Alcohol Problems Among the Unemployed." Current Alcohol Research 19 (1979):357-371.

Janis, Irving L. Short-Term Counseling: Guidelines Based on Recent Research. New Haven: Yale U. Press, 1983.

Jourard, Sidney M. The Transparent Self. New York: Van Nos. Reinhold, 1971.

Karoly, Paul and John J. Steffen, eds. Adolescent Behavior Disorders: Foundations and Contemporary Concerns. Vol. 3 Lexington, Mass: Lexington Books, 1984.

Keane, Anne, Joseph Ducette, and Diane C. Adler. "Stress in ICU and Non-ICU Nurses." Nursing Research 34 (1985):231-236.

Kemper, Theordore. A Social Interactional Theory. New York: John Wiley and Sons, 1984.

Kendall, Phillip C. Clinical Psychology. New York: John Wiley and Sons, 1984.

Kennison, Monica Metrick. "Faith: An Untapped Health Resource." Journal of Psychosocial Nursing 25 (1987):28-30.

Klerman, Gerald L. and Myrna M. Weissman. "Affective Responses to Stressful Life Events." Preventing Stress-Related Psychiatric Disorder eds. Howard H. Goldman and Stephen E. Goldston. Rockville, Maryland: National Institute of Mental Health, 1985:55-76

Kliman, Jodie, Rochelle Kern, and Ann Kliman. "Natural and Human-Made Disasters: Some Therapeutic and Epidemiological Implications for Crisis Intervention." Therapeutic Intervention: Healing Strategies for Human Services. eds. Uri Rueveni, Ross V. Speck, and Joan L. Speck. New York: Human Science Press, 1982:253-280.

Kobada, Suzanne C. "The Hardy Personality: Toward a Social Psychology of Stress and Health." Social Psychology of Health and Illness. eds. Glen S. Sanders and Jerry Suls. Hillsdale, New Jersey: Lawrence Erlbaum Associates, Publishers, 1982:3-32.

Kolditz, Doreen Anne and Rose Ann Naughton. Survival of Illness Implications for Nursing. New York: Springer Publishing Company, 1981.

Kubler-Ross, Elizabeth. Death, The Final Stage. New York: Prentice Hall, 1975.

Kuo, Wen H. and Tsai Yung-Mei. "Social Networking, Hardiness, and Immigrant's Mental Health." Journal of Health and Social Behavior 27 (1986):133-149.

L'Abate, Luciano. Systematic Family Therapy. New York: Brunner/Mazel, 1986.

L'Abate, Luciano, Gary Ganahl, and James C. Hansen. Methods of Family Therapy. Englewood Cliffs, New Jersey: Prentice Hall, 1986.

Lancaster, Jeanette and Wade Lancaster. "Current Status of the Health Care System" Community Health Nursing. eds. Marcia Stanhope and Jeanette Lancaster. St. Louis: C.V. Mosby Company, 1984:32-53.

Lasch, Christopher. The Minimal Self. New York: W. W. Norton, 1984.

Levine, Sol. "The Changing Terrains in Medical Sociology: Emergent Concerns with Quality of Life." Journal of Health and Social Behavior 28 (1987):1-6.

Levine, Sol and Marin A. Kozloff. "The Sick Role: Assessment and Overview." Annual Review Sociology 4 (1979):317-343.

Lifton, Robert Jay. The Broken Connection: On Death and the Continuity of Life. New York: Simon and Schuster, 1979.

Lin, Nan. "Epilogue: In Retrospect and Prospect." Social Support, Life Events,and Depression. eds. Nan Lin, Alfred Dean, and Walter M. Ensel. New York: Academic Press, 1986:333-362

Lin, Nan, Mary Woefel and Stephen C. Light. "Buffering the Impact of the Most Important Life Event." Social Support, Life Events, and Depression. eds. Nan Lin, Alfred Dean, and Walter M. Ensel. New York: Academic Press, 1986:307-332.

Lovinger, Robert J. Working with Religious Issues in Therapy. New York: Jason Aronson, 1984.

Lynch, James J. The Language of the Heart. New York: Basic Books, 1985.

McNall, Scott G. Theoretical Perspectives in Sociology. New York: St. Martin

Press, 1979.

MacManus, Susan A. "A Global View." Transaction: Social Science and Modern Society 23 (1986):51-53.

Maltsberger, John T. Suicide Risk: The Formulation of Clinical Judgment. New York: New York U. Press, 1986.

Marsella, Anthony J. and Georffrey M. White, eds. Cultural Conceptions of Mental Health and Therapy. Dordrecht: D. Reidel Publishing, 1984.

Maslach, Christina. "The Burnout Syndrome and Patient Care." Stress and Survival. ed. Charles A. Garfield. St. Louis: C. V. Mosby, 1979.

Maslow, Abraham. Motivation and Personality. New York: Harper and Row, 1954.

Matthews, Karen A. and Suzanne G. Haynes. "Type A Behavior Pattern and Coronary Disease Risk: Update and Critical Review." American Journal of Epidemiology 123 (1986):923-960.

Mattsson, Ake. "Long-Term Physical Illness in Childhood: A Challenge to Psychosocial Adaption." Stress and Survival. ed. Charles A. Garfield St. Louis: C. V. Mosby, 1979.

Melamed, Samuel. "Emotional Relativity and Elevated Blood Pressure." Psychosomatic Medicine 49 (1987):217-224.

Miles, Margaret Shandor. "Emotional Symptoms and Physical Health in Bereaved Parents." Nursing Research 134 (1985):76-81.

Miller, Patricia, Richard L. Wikoff, Margaret McMahon, Mary Jane Garrett, and Kathleen Ringel. "Indicators of Medical Regimen Adherence for Myocardial Infarction Patients." Nursing Research 34 (1985):268-272.

Morgan Gareth. "More on Metaphor: Why We Cannot Control Tropes." Administrative Science Quarterly 28 (1983):601-607.

Images of Organizations. Beverly Hills: Sage, 1986.

Muldary, Thomas W. Interpersonal Relations for Health Professionals: A Social Skills Approach. New York: Macmillan, 1983.

Social Skills Approach. New York: Macmillan, 1983.

Napodano, Rudolph J. Values in Medical Practice. New York: Human Sciences, 1986.

Norman, G. R., A. H. McFarlane, and D. L. Streiner. "Patterns of Illness Among Individuals Reporting High and Low Stress. Canadian Journal of Psychiatry 30 (1985):400-405.

Numerof, Rita E. The Practice of Management for Health Care Professionals. New York: American Management, 1982.

O'Hara, Delia. "Cancer Patients Flock to Mexican Clinic Despite Scientific Doubts." Chicago Sun Times, 3 September 1987.

Pamela V. Moore and Geraldine C. Williamson. "Health Promotion: Evolution of a Concept." Nursing Clinics of North America 19 (1984): 195-206.

Papadopoulos, Renos K. and Graham S. Saayman. Jung in Modern Perspective. Hounslow, Middlesex: Wildwood House, 1984.

Parker, Rolland S. Emotional Common Sense. Revised edition, 1973. New York: Harper and Row, 1981.

Purtilo, Ruth. Health Professional and Patient Interaction. 3rd ed. Philadelphia: W. B. Saunders, 1984.

Puryear, Douglas A. Helping People in Crisis. San Francisco: Jossey-Bass, 1979.

Rando, Therese A., ed. Loss and Anticipatory Grief. Lexington, Massachusetts: Lexington, 1986.

Reiner, Eckhart. "The Rehabilitation Team." Interdisciplinary Rehabilitation in Trauma. eds. John J. Gerhardt, Eckhart Reiner, Bernd Schwaiger, and Philip S. King. Baltimore: Williams and Wilkins, 1987:50-56.

Restak, Richard M. The Brain. New York: Bantam, 1984.

Rice, Joy K. and David G. Rice. Living Through Divorce. New York: The Guilford Press, 1986.

Richman, Joseph. Family Therapy for Suicidal People. New York: Springer, 1986.

Roger, Sylvia. "Parents as Therapists: A Responsible Alternative or Abrogation of Responsibility?" The Exceptional Child 33 (1986):17-27.

Rogers, Malcolm P. and Peter Reich. "Psychosomatic Medicine and Consultation-Liaison Psychiatry." The New Harvard Guide to Psychiatry. Cambridge: Harvard U. Press, 1988:387-417.

Rosellini, Gayle and Mark Worden. Of Course You're Angry. Central City, Minnesota: Hazelden Educational Materials, 1985.

Rueveni, Uri, Ross V. Speck, and Joan L. Speck, eds. Therapeutic Intervention: Healing Strategies for Human Systems. New York: Human Sciences Press, 1982.

Sanders, Glenn S. and Jerry Suls, eds. Social Psychology of Health and Illness. Hillsdale, New Jersey: Lawrence Erlbaum Associates, 1982.

Scheff, Thomas J. "Toward Integration in the Social Psychology of Emotions." Annual Review in Sociology 9 (1983):333-354.

Schlein, Stephen. A Way of Looking at Things. Selected Papers from 1930 to 1980 Erik H. Erikson. New York: W. W. Norton, 1987.

Schmolling, Paul, William Burger, and Merrill Youkeles. Helping People: A Guide to Careers in Mental Health. Englewood Cliffs, New Jersey: Prentice-Hall, 1981.

Schoenbach, Victor J., Berton H. Kaplan, Lisa Fredman, and David G. Kleinbaum. "Social Ties and Mortality in Evans County, Georgia." American Journal of Epidemiology 123 (1986):577-591.

Schoenberg, B. Mark, and Charles F. Preston, eds. Interactive Counseling. Westport, Connecticut: Greenwood, 1983.

Schultz, Susy. "60 % of Teen Moms Sexually Abused: Study." Chicago Sun Times, 15 September 1987.

Seltzer, Leon. Paradoxical Strategies in Psychotherapy. A Comprehensive Overview and Guidebook. New York: John Wiley and Sons, 1986.

Selye, Hans. The Stress of Life. New York: McGraw Hill, 1976.

Sennett, Richard. Authority. New York: Knopf, 1980.

Servan-Schreiber, Jean-Louis. The Return of Courage. Trans. Frances   Frenaye Reading, Massachusetts: Addison-Wesley, 1987.

Shapiro, Mary J. The Story of The Statue of Liberty and Ellis Island. New   York: Vintage, 1986.

Sidel, Victor W. and Ruth Sidel. Reforming Medicine: Lessons of the Past Quarter Century. New York: Pantheon, 1984.

Siegler, Miriam and Humphry Osmond. Patienthood: The Art of Being a Responsible Patient. New York: Macmillan, 1979.

Simpson, Richard L. Conferencing Parents of Exceptional Children. Rockville, Maryland: Aspen Publication, 1982.

Simross, Lynn. "Prevention Becomes 4th Revolution in Psychiatry." Los   Angeles Times, 17 September 1987

Slaby, Andrew Edmund and Arvin Sigmund Glicksman. Adapting to Life-Threatening Illness. New York: Praeger, 1985.

Slaikeu, Karl A. Crisis Intervention: A Handbook for Practice and Research. Boston: Allyn and Bacon, 1984.

Smart, R. G. "Drinking Problems Amongst Employed, Unemployed and Shift Workers." Journal of Medicine 21 (1979):731-736.

Smith, Anne. "The Brain Injured Patient: The Story of Brian."   Interdisciplinary Rehabilitation in Trauma. eds. John J. Gerhardt,   Echkhart Reiner, Bernd Schwaiger, and Philip King. Baltimore: Williams and Wilkins, 1987:3-9.

Smith, Dorothy W. Survival of Illness. New York: Springer, 1981.

Smith, G. Richard, Roberta A. Monson, and Debby C. Ray. "Psychiatric Consultation in Somatization Disorder." The New England Journal of Medicine 314 (1986):1407-1413.

Snook, I. Donald, Jr. and Leo D'Orazio. Opportunities in Health and Medical Careers. Lincolnwood, Illinois: National Textbook Company, 1984.

Stanhope, Marcia and Jeanette Lancaster, eds. Community Health Nursing. St. Louis: The C. V. Mosby, 1984.

Stark, Werner. The Social Bond, Vol.2. New York: Fordham U. Press, 1978.

Steele, Robert S. Freud and Jung. Boston: Routledge, 1982.

Stinnett, Nick and John DeFain. Secrets of Strong Families. New York: Little Brown, 1986.

Strubreither, Wilheim. "Psychology." Interdisciplinary Rehabilitation in Trauma. eds. John J. Gerhardt, Echkhart Reiner, Bernd Schwaiger, and Philip King. Baltimore: Williams and Wilkins, 1987:212-215.

Stryker, Sheldon. Symbolic Interactionism: A Structural Version. Menlo Park, California: The Benjamin/Cummings Publishing Company, 1980.

Sugarman, Stuart. The Family Therapy Collections. Rockville, Maryland: An Aspen Publication, 1986.

Talbott, John A. "Community Psychiatry." The Year Book of Psychiatry and Applied Mental Health. eds. Daniel X. Freeman, Reginald S. Lourie, Herbert Y. Meltzer, John C. Nemiah, John A. Talbott, and Herbert Weiner Chicago: Year Book Medical Publishers, 1987:391-467.

Terhune, James. "Teaching Skills for Healthy Lifestyles." Health Education (1986):4-7.

Trotter, Robert J. "Stop Blaming Yourself." Psychology Today 21 (1987): 31-38.

Turner, Jonathan H. "Toward a Sociological Theory of Motivation." American Sociological Review 52 (1987):15-27.

Unger, Roberto Mangabeira. Passions. New York: The Free Press, 1986.

Vash, Carolyn L. "Quality of Life Issues Affecting People with Disabilities." Public Policy Issues Impacting the Future of Rehabilitation in America.

ed. William G. Emener. Stillwater, Oklahoma: National Clearing House of Rehabilitation Training Materials, 1987:2-35.

Veninga, Robert L. A Gift of Hope: How We Survive Our Tragedies. New York:Ballantine, 1986.

Viney L. L. and A. M. Clarke. "A General Systems Approach to the Patient, Hospital Staff, Family, and Community: Implications for Health Care Services." Behavioral Science 31 (1986):239-253.

Viorst, Judith Necessary Losses. New York: Simon and Schuster, 1986.

Wagner, Roy. Symbols That Stand for Themselves. Chicago: The U. of Chicago Press, 1986.

Walker, J. Ingram. Psychiatric Emergencies Intervention and Resolution. Philadelphia: J.B. Lippincott, 1983.

Weary, Gifford and Herbert L. Mirels. Integration of Clinical and Social Psychology. Oxford: Oxford U. Press, 1982.

Weiner, Herbert. "Psychosomatic Medicine." The Year Book of Psychiatry and Applied Mental Health. eds. Daniel X. Freedman, Reginald S. Lourie, Herbert Y. Meltzer, John C. Nemiah, John A. Talbott, and Herbert Weiner Chicago: Year Book Medical Publishers, 1987:199-200.

Weinstein, Kate. Living with Endometriosis. Reading, Massachusetts:Addison-Wesley Publishing, 1987.

Weizman, Savine Gross and Phyllis Kamm. About Mourning: Support and Guidance for the Bereaved. New York: Human Sciences Press, 1985.

Wethington, Elaine and Ronald C. Kessler. "Perceived Support, Received Support, and Adjustment to Stressful Life Events." Journal of Health and Social Behavior 27 (1986):78-89.

Wheaton, Blair. "Models for the Stress-Buffering Functions of Coping Resources." Journal of Health and Social Behavior 26 (1985):352-364.

Wile, Daniel B. Couple Therapy: A Nontraditional Approach. New York: John Wiley and Sons, 1981.

Wilson J. "Patients' Wants Versus Patients' Interest." Journal of Medical Ethics 12 (1986):127-132.

Windholz, Michael J., Charles R. Marmar, and Mardi J. Horowitz. "A Review of the Research on Conjugal Bereavement: Impact of Health and Efficacy of Intervention." Comprehensive Psychiatry 26 (1985):433-447.

Woodson, Robert. "Hospice Care in Terminal Illness." Stress and Survival. ed. Charles A. Garfield. St. Louis: C. V. Mosby, 1979.

Yuker, H. "Attitudes Toward the Disabled." Disability: Our Challenge. ed. J. Hourihan. New York: Columbia Teachers College, 1979.

Yuker, H. and J. Block. Research with the Attitude Toward Disabled Persons Scale 1960-1985. Hempstead, New York: Hofstra U. Center for the Study of Attitudes Toward Persons with Disability, 1987.

INDEX